Official Journal of the European Societ

AF887677

International Journal of

Microcirculation

Clinical and Experimental

Founded 1980 by the European Society for Microcirculation

KARGER

Printed in Switzerland
on acid-free paper by
Thür AG Offsetdruck, Pratteln

Appears bimonthly:
1 volume per year (6 issues)

International Journal of
Microcirculation
Clinical and Experimental

International Journal of Microcirculation publishes manuscripts of scientific excellence in microvascular research and vascular biology. Manuscripts may be in the form of research papers, reviews, rapid communications and correspondence.

Submission: Only original manuscripts written in English are considered. Research papers and reviews should not normally be more than 10 printed pages in length including illustrations and references (6,460 characters per page). Authors wishing to submit a review should contact the Editors in advance. Rapid communications should not exceed 3 printed pages. Correspondence and Commentary should be brief. Manuscripts should be sent to the Editors-in-Chief:

Prof. Dr. K. Messmer
Institute for Surgical Research
University of Munich
Marchioninistrasse 15
D–81366 München (FRG)
Tel. 89-7095 4400
Fax 89-7095 8897

Clinical papers to:

Doc. Dr. B. Fagrell
Karolinska Institute
Department of Medicine
Karolinska Sjukhuset
S–171 76 Stockholm (Sweden)
Tel. 46-8-7295402
Fax 46-8-344293

To facilitate a rapid review process, authors are asked to supply their telephone and fax numbers.

Manuscripts, including photocopies of line drawings, should be submitted in quadruplicate, typewritten double-spaced on one side of the paper, 10 characters per inch, with a margin not less than 25 mm on each side. Two photographs of line-drawings and four copies of micrographs should be supplied on glossy paper.

Conditions: All manuscripts are subject to editorial review. Manuscripts are received with the explicit understanding that they are not under simultaneous consideration by any other publication. Submission of an article for publication implies the transfer of the copyright from the author to the publisher upon acceptance. Accepted papers become the permanent property of 'International Journal of Microcirculation' and may not be reproduced by any means, in whole or in part, without the written consent of the publisher. It is the author's responsibility to obtain permission to reproduce illustrations, tables, etc. from other publications.

Arrangement of Research papers

Manuscript organization: Manuscripts should include, in sequence and on separate pages: title and authors, address, running title and acknowledgment of support; abstract and key words; introduction; methods; results; discussion; acknowledgments; references; tables; figures. The normal maximum length is 10 printed pages (including tables, illustrations and references), one printed page containing 6,460 letters, spaces included.

Title page: The first page of each paper should indicate the title (main title underlined), the authors' names, and the institute where the work was conducted. A short title for use as running head is also required.

Full address: The exact postal address complete with postal code of the senior author must be given. To expedite the review process, telephone and fax numbers should be provided. If correspondence is handled by someone else, indicate this accordingly.

Key words: For indexing purposes, a list of 3 – 10 key words in English is essential.

Abstract: Each paper needs an abstract of up to 200 words.

Style: Use generic names of drugs. Avoid jargon, euphemisms and abbreviations.

Small type: Paragraphs which can or must be set in smaller type (case histories, test methods, etc.) should be indicated with a 'p' (petit) in the margin on the left-hand side.

Footnotes: Acknowledgment of support is printed as a footnote to the title. Other footnotes should be avoided. When essential, they are numbered consecutively and typed at the foot of the appropriate page.

Tables and illustrations: Tables and illustrations (both numbered in Arabic numerals) should be prepared on separate sheets. Tables require a heading and figures a legend, also prepared on a separate sheet. For the reproduction of illustrations, only good drawings and original photographs can be accepted; negatives or photocopies cannot be used. Due to technical reasons, figures with a screen background should not be submitted. When possible, group several illustrations on one block for reproduction (max. size 181 × 223 mm) or provide crop marks. On the back of each illustration, indicate its number, the author's name, and 'top' with a soft pencil.

Color illustrations: Up to 6 color illustrations per page can now be integrated with the text at the reduced price of CHF 600.– / USD 545.00 per page. Color illustrations are reproduced at the author's expense.

References: In the text identify references by Arabic numerals [in square brackets]. Material submitted for publication but not yet accepted should be noted as 'unpublished data' and not be included in the reference list. The list of references should include only those publications which are cited in the text. Do not alphabetize; number references in the order in which they are first mentioned in the text. The surnames of the authors followed by initials should be given. There should be no punctuation other than a comma to separate the authors. Cite all authors, 'et al' is not sufficient. Abbreviate journal names according to the Index Medicus system. (Also see International Committee of Medical Journal Editors: Uniform requirements for manuscripts submitted to biomedical journals. Br Med J 1988;296:401–405.)

Examples

(a) Papers published in periodicals: Shirahase H, Fujiwara M, Usui H, Kurahashi K: A possible role of thromboxane A_2 in endothelium in maintaining resting tone and producing contractile response to acetylcholine and arachidonic acid in canine cerebral arteries. Blood Vessels 1987;24:117–119.

(b) Monographs: Matthews DE, Farewell VT: Using and Understanding Medical Statistics. Basel, Karger, 1985.

(c) Edited books: Duling BR, Sleek GE: Mechanical aspects of endothelial cell–smooth muscle cell interactions in resistance vessels; in Bevan JA, Majewski H, Maxwell RH, Story DF (eds): Vascular Neuroeffector Mechanisms. Oxford, IRL Press, 1988, pp 23–30.

Further details: Authors may consult our leaflet 'Rules for the Preparation of Manuscripts', available on request from the Publisher, S. Karger AG, P.O. Box, CH – 4009 Basel (Switzerland).

Rapid communication: Manuscripts intended for rapid communication must present new findings of sufficient importance to justify their accelerated acceptance. They should follow the general arrangement of research papers. No abstracts or introduction is required, but the first paragraph should include the reason for the study and the main findings. They should not be more than three printed pages in length (including figures, tables and references). Proofs are checked by the Main Editor and not sent to the authors. Review will be rapid, and once accepted, the paper will be included in the next planned issue.

Reviews: Reviews concerned with topics in vascular research of current interest will be welcomed. Potential authors are asked to check first with the Editors to avoid clashes with other pending reviews. All reviews will be subjected to normal critical peer refereeing.

Correspondence: Letters to the Editor concerning articles published in International Journal of Microcirculation may be submitted for publication. If accepted, the authors of the articles concerned will be given the opportunity to reply.

Commentary: Comments concerning current topics of interest in vascular science will be considered for publication by the Editors. They should not be more than one printed page.

Galley proofs: Unless indicated otherwise, galley proofs are sent to the first-named author and should be returned with the least possible delay. Alterations made in galley proofs, other than the correction of printer's errors, are charged to the author. No page proofs are supplied.

Reprints: The main authors of all papers appearing in Volumes 14 and 15 will receive a one-year subscription and 50 reprints free of charge. Order forms and a price list are sent with the galley proofs. Orders submitted after the issue is printed are subject to considerably higher prices. Allow five weeks from the date of publication for delivery.

KARGER

General Information

International Journal of **Microcirculation** Clinical and Experimental

Publication data: 'International Journal of Microcirculation' is published 6 times annually. Volume 15 with 6 issues appears in 1995.

Subscription rates: Subscriptions run for a full calendar year. Prices are given per volume.

Personal subscription:

Subscription + postage and handling
SFr. 349.30 + SFr. 17.90 Europe
SFr. 349.30 + SFr. 27.30 Overseas
US$ 268.80 + US$ 17.90
(Must be in the name of, billed to, and paid by an individual. Order must be marked 'personal subscription'.)

Institutional subscription:

Subscription + postage and handling
SFr. 499.– + SFr. 25.50 Europe
SFr. 499.– + SFr. 39.– Overseas
US$ 384.00 + US$ 25.50

Airmail postage: SFr. 36.–, US$ 30.00. (Extra per volume.)

Microforms: Please direct all enquiries and orders to:
University Microfilms Inc.
300 North Zeeb Road, P.O. Box 1346
Ann Arbor, MI 48106-1346 (USA)

Subscription orders: Orders can be placed at agencies, bookstores, directly with the Publisher S. Karger AG, P.O. Box, CH–4009 Basel (Switzerland) or with any of the following distributors:

Deutschland: S. Karger GmbH, Postfach D–79095 Freiburg
France: Librairie Luginbühl 36, bd de Latour-Maubourg, F–75007 Paris
Great Britain, Ireland: S. Karger Publishers 11 Ravenscroft Road Beckenham, Kent BR3 4TP
USA: S. Karger Publishers, Inc. 26 West Avon Road, P.O. Box 529 Farmington, CT 06085
India, Bangladesh, Sri Lanka: S. Karger India Subscription Agency B–5/132 Safdarjung Enclave New Delhi-110029
Japan: Katakura Libri, Inc. Take 1 Bldg, 2nd Floor, 4-5-7 Yushima Bunkyo-ku, Tokyo 113

Change of address: Both old and new address should be sent to the subscription source.

Advertising: Correspondence and rate requests should be addressed to the Publisher.

Single issues and back volumes: Information can be obtained through the Publisher.

Bibliographic indices: This journal is regularly listed in bibliographic services.

KARGER

Functional Capillary Density: Active and Passive Determinants

Satellite Symposium to the Meeting of the Microcirculatory Society, Newport Beach, Calif., April 22, 1994

Guest Editors
Marcos Intaglietta, La Jolla, Calif.
Paul C. Johnson, Tucson, Ariz.

43 figures, 4 tables, 1995

KARGER

S. Karger
Medical and Scientific Publishers
Basel · Freiburg · Paris · London
New York · New Delhi · Bangkok
Singapore · Tokyo · Sydney

Drug Dosage
The authors and the publisher have exerted every effort to ensure that drug selection and dosage set forth in this text are in accord with current recommendations and practice at the time of publication. However, in view of ongoing research, changes in government regulations, and the constant flow of information relating to drug therapy and drug reactions, the reader is urged to check the package insert for each drug for any change in indications and dosage and for added warnings and precautions. This is particularly important when the recommended agent is a new and/or infrequently employed drug.

Printed in Switzerland on acid-free paper by
Thür AG Offsetdruck, Pratteln
ISBN 3-8055-6288-8

Contents

Int J Microcirc 1995;15:217

M. Intaglietta, La Jolla, Calif.
P.C. Johnson, Tucson, Ariz.

Introduction

Capillaries are historically the final entry in the description of the organic components of the cardiovascular system. Correspondingly, a precise understanding of their function and behavior has been late in developing and surprisingly is not yet complete. Although we are rapidly advancing in our knowledge of the molecular basis of cellular processes, the structure, behavior and function of this most extensive and ubiquitous organ system, spanning about 1,000 km per kilogram of tissue, remain elusive.

Capillaries, first envisioned as the connection between the arteries and veins, became conceptually locked as entities functioning to convey oxygen, a process modulated by the blood stream factors of oxygenation, oxygen carrying capacity, and blood flow velocity. Although it was recognized from the very beginning, that there was a natural variability in the number and frequency of capillaries with red blood cell passage, no systematic attempts were made to determine the mechanism underlying the fluctuations in the number of capillaries with blood flow. Failure to identify an anatomical 'precapillary sphincter' and the notion that capillaries were relatively rigid structures endowed the capillary system with a static permanence, and the mechanism regulating blood throughput became assigned to the arterioles.

The laissez faire surrounding capillaries is exemplified by our concepts of 'capillary recruitment' in the analysis of muscle perfusion during exercise. In this context, it became well established that increased metabolic demand was satisfied by an increased number of conduits convecting blood through the tissue, but little attention was given to the state and conditions of these conduits when the demand was not present.

The recognition of the existence of reperfusion injury and 'no-reflow' phenomena caused capillaries to return to the limelight as entities with autonomous properties that in given circumstances could become transiently or permanently impaired. 'Functional capillary density' has now become a variable describing how the tissue will fare when it is subjected to stress. The increased use of this term and the recognition that its variability has diverse origins led us to organize a symposium to address mechanisms that affect tissue perfusion at the level of single capillaries.

The contributions to this Symposium highlight the fact that control of single capillary perfusion has many components. Mechanically it is determined by the interaction between the formed elements of blood and the geometrical features of the conduits. Biochemical events in the endothelium are a primary determinant of flow in pathophysiological conditions, and the interaction between hydraulic and osmotic pressure in modulating tissue volume and capillary dimensions affect the dimensions of the capillary structure as a whole. Furthermore, there is increasing evidence that there may be a form of single-capillary vasomotion originating from spontaneous activity in endothelial cells. This limited enumeration of flow effectors leads to speculation about the signals to which capillaries respond and whether oxygen and other metabolites may be determinants of flow modulation in single units. It remains an open question as to what is a 'closed' capillary and the events that occur in its environment in this condition.

As a historical note, this symposium 'Functional Capillary Density: Active and Passive Determinants' was held in Huntington Beach, Calif., USA, April 22, 1994. It is the last of a series of symposia held over the past decade in conjunction with the annual meeting of the Microcirculatory Society, and sponsored by the Tucson-San Diego-Baltimore Program Project on Regulation and Exchange in the Microcirculation supported by NIH grant HL17421. Unification of two laboratories in this Program Project brought by the move of P.C. Johnson to San Diego and evolution of the experimental research program now housed in a single institution in one city will undoubtedly lead to new opportunities for the continuation of this forum on research and study of the microcirculation.

Int J Microcirc 1995;15:218–222

P.C. Johnson

Department of Physiology, University of Arizona, Tucson, Ariz., USA

Active and Passive Determinants of Capillary Density: A Historical Perspective

Key Words
Capillary density
Regulation
Shunts

Abstract
Capillary density has historically been an important issue, beginning with the discovery of the circulation and extending to the present day. Determination of capillary density provided key evidence supporting the concept that the entire cardiac output passed through microscopic channels in the tissue and returned to the heart. Subsequently, control of capillary density by contractility of the capillaries themselves was proposed by Krogh. Later investigators disputed the notion of capillary contractility and proposed that changes in capillary density were secondary to changes in arteriolar tone or to passive mechanical factors. While this is still the prevailing view, the concept that the capillaries are not totally passive and may, through shape changes of the endothelia, alter the distribution of flow through the capillary network is under active consideration. While views of underlying mechanism vary, there is agreement that capillary density and its control are of fundamental importance to our understanding of the function of the microcirculation.

A historical view of the determinants of capillary density may logically begin with those who first observed capillaries, most notably Anton van Leeuwenhoek (fig. 1a), who described in 1674 the capillary network in the tail of the eel, as shown in fig. 1b. van Leeuwenhoek's observations [2] provided direct evidence for the existence of what Harvey referred to as invisible 'porosities of the flesh' through which blood flowed from the left to the right side of the heart. van Leeuwenhoek's studies also addressed one of the main objections to Harvey's theory, namely, that is seemed unlikely that the large volume of blood said to be expelled from the heart with each beat could pass through such small channels.

To answer this objection, van Leeuwenhoek made the first measurements of capillary density, meticulously counting the number of capillaries in a cirumscribed region of the tail fin of the eel. Armed with this information, he argued on a quantitive basis that if such a small tissue area contained so many capillaries, then it was not illogical that the entire body would indeed have a sufficient number of capillaries to accept the entire cardiac output postulated by Harvey. Thus the measurement of capillary density provided critical evidence in support of Harvey's theory of the circulation of the blood.

The question of whether capillary density is a fixed or variable quantity was subsequently addressed by Krogh.

Paul C. Johnson
Department of Bioengineering
University of California San Diego
La Jolla, CA 92093-0412 (USA)

0167–6865/95/0155–0218
$10.00/0

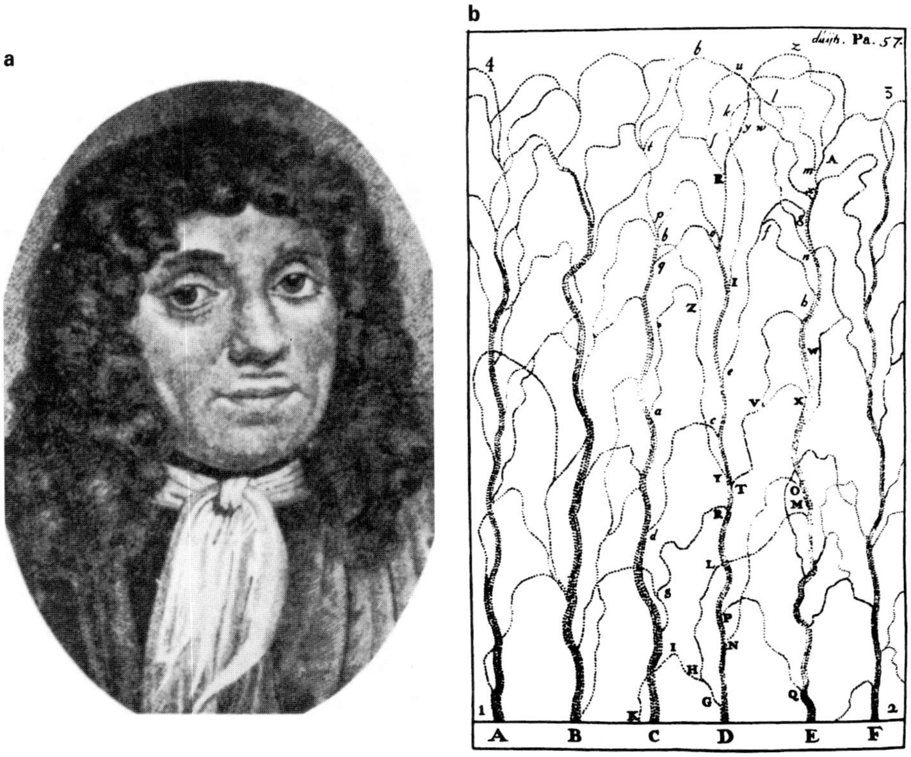

Fig. 1. a Anton van Leeuwenhoek. **b** The microvascular network of the tail of the eel as described by van Leeuwenhoek. Reproduced from Landis [1], with permission.

In his classic Silliman lectures at Yale 1922 [3], Krogh described studies in which an extract of posterior pituitary appeared to cause contraction of capillaries in the frog tongue. He also emphasized the importance of capillary density and its regulation [4]. In his view, it would be a wasteful expenditure of energy to perfuse all the capillaries simultaneously except during periods of high oxygen demand. This was based on studies in which he injected India ink into the circulation of the frog, sacrified the animal, and examined the distribution of the ink in the capillary network of skeletal muscles. In resting muscle, ink was found in only a small percentage of the capillaries while in exercising muscle it was present in virtually all capillaries.

On the basis of these observations, he proposed that capillary density is a regulated variable, with individual capillaries opening and closing according to local metabolic conditions as shown in figure 2. This, he suggested, was due to the intrinsic contractility of Rouget cells or pericytes adjacent to the capillaries. These experiments may have been flawed by the tendency of the ink particles to aggregate, and thus at low flows the number of capillaries with blood flow may have been underestimated. A more direct challenge to the active capillary theory was presented by investigators such as Zweifach [5] in 1937 in studies on capillaries of frog mesentery and Clark and

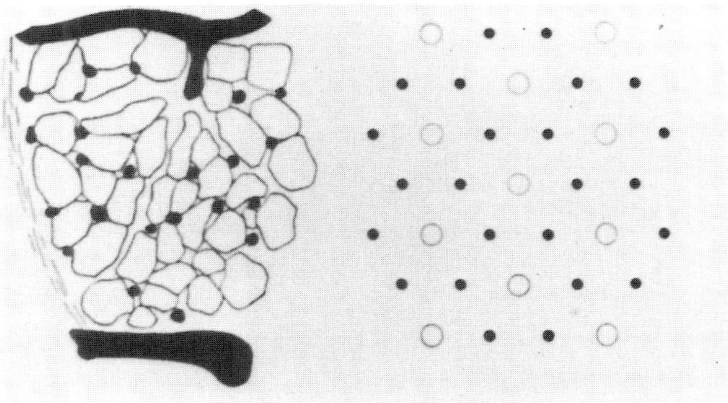

Fig. 2. Krogh's concept of open and closed capillaries which changed in an alternating pattern to supply blood to each capillary for a limited period of time. Reproduced from Landis [2], with permission.

Clark [6] in the early 1940s in studies of capillaries in the ear chamber of the rabbit. Both laboratories were unable to confirm that capillaries possess the ability to contract. However, the concept of regulation of capillary density has been an enduring one based on other studies as well.

With the growth of knowledge of the microcirculation, mechanisms other than contraction of individual capillaries were proposed for regulating capillary density. Fore-

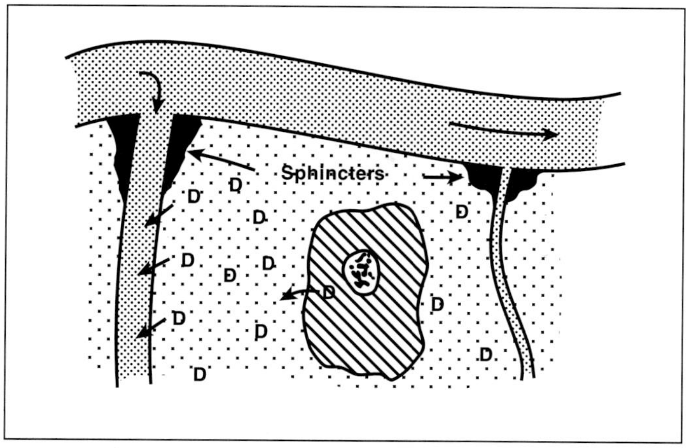

Fig. 3. The concept of separate control of perfusion through individual capillaries by precapillary sphincters. From Winsor and Hyman [8], with permission.

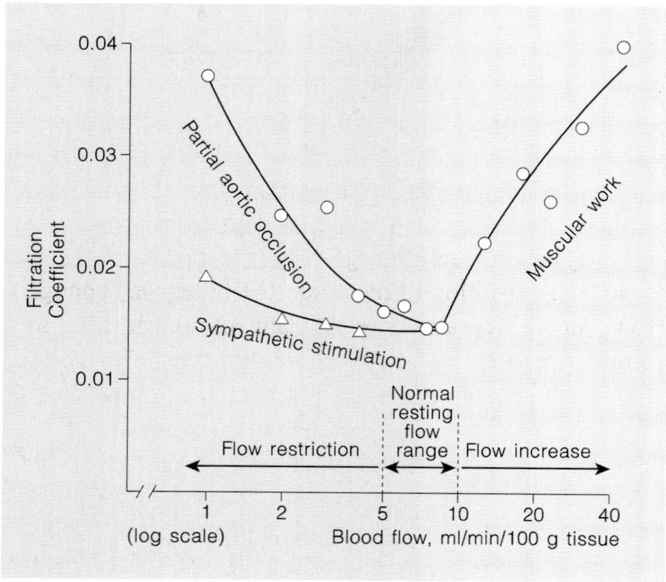

Fig. 4. Relation between capillary filtration coefficient and blood flow in skeletal muscle. Note that both increase and decrease in blood flow are accompanied by an increase in the filtration coefficient, indicating that capillary surface area is controlled separately from blood flow. From Cobbold et al. [10], with permission.

most among these is the precapillary sphincter, whose contractile properties were described, among others, by Fulton and Lutz [7]. The precapillary sphincter, located at the entrance to individual capillaries, was said to possess a degree of intrinsic tone which could effectively close the entrance to the capillary lumen. However, in response to an accumulation of local vasodilator metabolites, Winsor and Hyman [8] suggested the entrance would open as shown in figure 3. Thus, the precapillary sphincter was envisioned as the means of adjusting capillarry density in accordance with metabolic requirements of the tissue.

The concept of physiological regulation of capillary density received additional support from whole organ studies in which resistance to blood flow and capillary exchange could be independently measured and compared. Folkow and coworkers reported extensively on vascular resistance and capillary filtration coefficient in skin, skeletal muscle and intestine under a variety of physiological conditions [9]. Changes in capillary filtration coefficient were thought to reflect alterations in the amount of capillary surface area available for exchange, which in turn was attributed to alteration in the number of capillaries with blood flow. In such studies, it was found in many instances that blood flow and exchange surface area appeared to change in the same direction, as would be expected if precapillary resistance vessels were controlling the number of capillaries with blood flow. For example, in figure 4, the capillary filtration coefficient increases as flow increases in skeletal muscle during muscle contraction [10]. But this is not always the case as also shown in figure 4, since the capillary filtration coefficient also increases when flow falls during sympathetic nerve stimulation. The latter finding supports the concept of separate regulation of available capillary exchange surface and vascular resistance. Using measurements of rate of loss of diffusible indicators, Renkin [11] and others assessed the combined permeability and vascular surface area available for diffusional exchange, the PS product. Renkin noted that the time course of change of the PS product did not always correlate with that of vascular resistance during muscle contraction.

In view of the disparity between apparent changes in available exchange surface and resistance of precapillary vessels, it was proposed that the precapillary sphincter was responsible for adjusting flow distribution in the capillary bed and that control of these elements was, to some extent, separate from the control of the arterioles [10]. For example, to explain the findings shown in Figure 4 during sympathetic nerve stimulation, it was suggested that the response to vasodilator metabolites was more pronounced in the sphincters than in the arterioles, the latter being under a greater degree of neural control than the sphincters.

While the precapillary sphincter provided an explanation for disparity between changes in vascular resistance and exchange, microcirculatory studies in certain key vas-

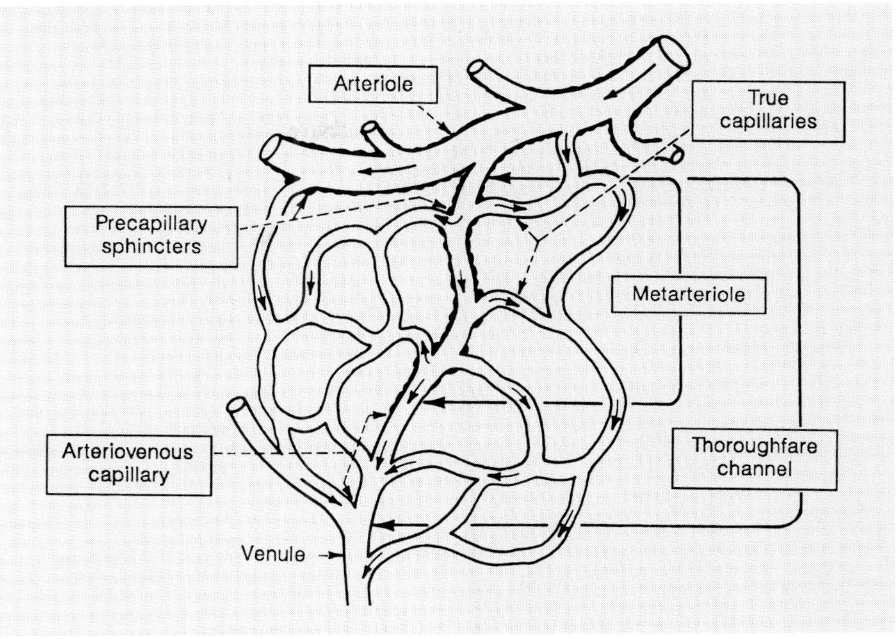

Fig. 5. A schematic of the mesenteric microcirculation. From Friedman [15], with permission.

cular beds such as skeletal muscle failed to confirm the existence of such structures [10]. The absence of explicit evidence for sphincters did not however rule out the possiblility that other precapillary vessels such as the terminal arterioles might perform the same function as attributed to the sphincter with flow through a group of capillaries being controlled by a single terminal arteriole.

A second possibility for varying capillary density that has been proposed is a passive adjustment of flow through parallel channels. According to this concept, deformation of the formed elements of the blood requires expenditure of energy and at low flows the pressure gradient across the capillary network is insufficient in some fraction of the capillaries [12]. In this instance, one would expect a direct relation between capillary density and blood flow seen during muscle contraction as shown in figure 4, but not the inverse relation seen during aortic occlusion. Microcirculatory studies have shown that the number of capillaries with flow stasis can increase considerably during reduced flow brought about by lowering arterial pressure or increasing vascular tone. Recent studies of morphological changes in endothelial cells described in this symposium raise the possibility that shape changes of these cells could influence flow distribution in capillary neworks.

Another concept that has been tied to the issue of capillary density is arteriovenous shunts. Friedman [13] proposed that the function of such shunts was to adjust the exchange surface area independently of flow by allowing some of the blood to pass through vessels which did not permit free diffusional exchange across the vessel wall. Evidence in favor of such a mechanism was based on a disparity between exchange of diffusible indicators as compared with blood flow when the latter was changed. However, thick-walled vessels connecting arterioles and venules are rare except in a few specialized vascular beds such as the tongue and skin [11]. Possibly contributing to functional shunting in certain circumstances would be the presence of channels such as the thoroughfare channel of the mesentery shown in figure 5. As first described by Chambers and Zweifach [14], the thoroughfare channel has a somewhat larger diameter and greater volume flow than do vessels emanating from this channel. The latter are sometimes referred to as 'true capillaries'. In vascular beds such as skeletal muscle where functional shunting is observed with indicator techniques, in vivo network studies have failed to reveal thoroughfare channels [11], indicating that functional shunting may occur in a network of vessels that appear morphologically similar. Interpretation of whole organ findings has, however, tended to rely on morphologically different pathways, without taking sufficient account of the wide range of flows in capillaries and the variable nature of capillary flow, the causes of which are currently under investigation.

In summary, quantitative assessment of capillary density has been an important issue since the discovery of the circulation over 350 years ago. In this century attention has been directed primarily toward measuring functional capillary density and understanding the mechanisms that determine it during physiological perturbations. Recently, as is evident in this symposium, there has been growing interest in functional capillary density in pathophysiological states and the special factors that may play a role under these conditions. Given the critical function that the capillaries perform in maintaining tissue homeostasis, better understanding of the determinants of functional capillary density will no doubt continue to be as important in the future as it has been in the past.

References

1 Landis EM: The capillary circulation; in Circulation of the Blood; A History of Men and Ideas. Bethesda, American Physiological Society, 1964, pp 355–406.

2 van Leeuwenhoek A: Select Works, Containing his Microscopical Discoveries in Many of the Works of Nature (Samuel Hook, trans). London, Nicol, 1964;1798–1807, vol 1, p 89.

3 Krogh A: The Anatomy and Physiology of Capillaries. New Haven, Yale University Press, 1929.

4 Krogh A: Reminiscences of work on capillary circulation. Isis 1950;41:14.

5 Zweifach BW: The structure and reactions of small blood vessels in amphibia. Am J Anat 1937;60:473–514.

6 Clark ER, Clark EL: Caliber changes in minute blood vessels observed in the living mammal. Am J Anat 1943;73:215–250.

7 Fulton GP, Lutz BR: The control of small blood vessels. Am J Physiol 1941;133:284.

8 Winsor T, Hyman C: A Primer of Peripheral Vascular Diseases. Philadelphia, Lea and Febiger, 1965, p 67.

9 Folkow B, Mellander S: Measurement of capillary filtration coefficient and its use in studies of the control of capillary exchange; in Crone C, Lasser NA (eds): Capillary Permeability. Copenhagen, Munksgaard, 1970, pp 614–623.

10 Cobbold A, Folkow B, Kjellmer I, Mellander S: Nervous and chemical control of precapillary sphincters in skeletal muscle as measured by changes in filtration coefficient. Acta Physiol Scand 1963;57:180–192.

11 Renkin E: Control of the microcirculation and blood-tissue exchange; in Handbook of Physiology, section 2: The Cardiovascular System. Vol IV: Microcirculation, part 2. Bethesda, American Physiological Society, 1984, pp 626–688.

12 Lindbom L, Arfors KE: Mechanisms and site of control for variation in the number of perfused capillaries in skeletal muscle. Int J Microcirc Clin Exp 1985;4:19–30.

13 Friedman JJ: Single passage extraction of ^{86}Rb from the circulation of skeletal muscle. Am J Physiol 1969;216:460–466.

14 Chambers R, Zweifach BW: Topography and function of the mesenteric capillary circulation. Am J Anat 1944;75:173–205.

15 Friedman JJ: Microcirculation; in Selkurt EE (ed): Physiology, ed 3. Boston, Little, Brown, 1971, ch 12.

Int J Microcirc 1995;15:223–230

A.C. Groom[a, b]
C.G. Ellis[a, b]
S.J. Wrigley[a]
R.F. Potter[a, b]

[a] Department of Medical Biophysics, University of Western Ontario, and
[b] The Colonel Tom Lawson Family Microcirculation Laboratory, John P. Robarts Research Institute, London, Ont., Canada

Capillary Network Morphology and Capillary Flow

Key Words
Capillary network structure/function
Skeletal muscle microcirculation
Capillary hemodynamics/RBC flow
Spatial heterogeneity
Temporal heterogeneity
RBC flow redistribution

Abstract

This paper examines the authors' research on capillary network morphology and the heterogeneity of capillary red cell (RBC) perfusion in skeletal muscle with the aim of demonstrating that capillary network structure plays a major role in determining flow distribution. Capillary network morphology was examined by quantifying the heterogeneity of capillary diameters, path and segment lengths, as well as the changes in configuration that occur as vessels accommodate themselves to continual changes of fiber length. Because of the network complexity and the two-phase nature of the perfusing blood, both *spatial* (i.e. among capillaries) and *temporal* heterogeneity of capillary perfusion were predicted to result. By means of computer analysis of video images of the microcirculation in vivo, we have demonstrated that more than 70% of the total spatial heterogeneity of capillary RBC perfusion arises from the capillary network as opposed to the arterioles, and that RBC flow continuously redistributes among capillaries. The spatial heterogeneity increases substantially as the arteriolar input to the network falls, and the data predict that during low-flow states, the network will fail to distribute blood properly among its constituent vessels. Thus passive rheological mechanisms and capillary network morphology are important determinants of functional capillary density.

Capillary dimensions and the branching nature of the capillary network have important implications for red blood cell (RBC) flow in capillaries. The extent of capillary interconnections in a network ranges from maximal in respiratory organs such as lung, or the chorioallantoic membrane of avian embryos, to zero in the rete mirabile of the eel. The network in lung has even been described as a 'sheet flow' system, whereas the eel rete consists of straight, unbranched capillaries almost 5 mm in length. We have some knowledge of the capillary network in a number of organs and tissues, but nowhere has this been studied in such detail as in skeletal muscle. This paper focuses on network morphology and RBC flow within the capillary bed of skeletal muscle.

In the context of active and passive determinants of functional capillary density, we must recognize that there are two major determinants of capillary flow distribution, the arteriolar network and the capillary network itself. The arteriolar network structure (fig. 1) may be revealed by partial perfusion of the microvasculature with Microfil [1]. Each terminal arteriole gives rise to a capillary network (fig. 2) which includes several divergent and convergent bifurcations before merging with the collecting venule [2]. By altering vascular tone to induce either vasoconstriction or vasodilatation, the arteriolar network can adjust the total blood flow to the muscle, whereas by altering the tone of selected terminal arterioles, the network can alter the distribution of blood flow to particular

Dr. Alan C. Groom
Department of Medical Biophysics
Health Sciences Centre
University of Western Ontario
London, Ontario N6A 5C1 (Canada)

0167–6865/95/0155–0223
$10.00/0

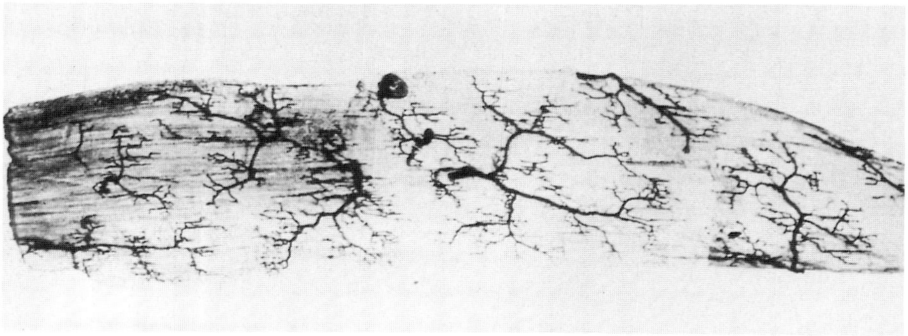

Fig. 1. Composite photomicrograph showing the undersurface of a frog sartorius muscle 27 mm in length, in which only the arterial vascular system has been perfused with an opaque silicone elastomer, Microfil. The structure of each arteriolar network may be seen down to the level of the capillaries, which Microfil has just begun to enter. From Plyley [1].

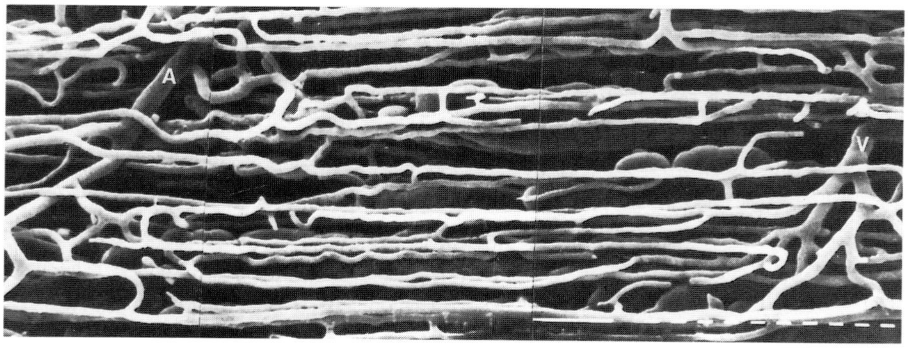

Fig. 2. Scanning electron micrograph (composite) taken at surface of microvascular corrosion cast from gastrocnemius muscle of rat. The limb was immobilized with the muscle at full extension, in situ. Section of the capillary network showing its associated arteriolar (A) and venular (V) trees. Short bars = 10 μm. From Groom et al. [2].

groups of capillaries. However, even if arteriolar flow were homogeneous, there would still be heterogeneity of capillary flow, because of the structure of the capillary network. This forms the focus of the present paper.

Capillary Morphology

Individual capillaries are irregular tubes fabricated from endothelial cells attached to a basement membrane, the luminal diameter being smaller than the lengths or widths of the cells and intrinsically irregular, due to variations in configuration among endothelial cells. At several positions along a capillary, the nuclear regions of endothelial cells can be seen bulging into the lumen (fig. 3), giving rise to narrowings of the vessel. These are not necessarily static features, for in some organs (e.g. spleen, pancreas), dynamic changes occur either spontaneously or in response to norepinephrine [3–6].

Changes in luminal cross section along a capillary give rise to changes in mean flow velocity with axial position [7–9], such that at points only 100 μm apart, there may be a difference of 50% or more in mean RBC velocity. Even more important, severe restrictions of luminal cross section may make it difficult or impossible for RBCs and leukocytes to pass along the capillary [4]. Theoretical studies have indicated that even the presence of several less severe luminal constrictions along a capillary may be sufficient to block the passage of RBCs at lower driving pressures [10], reducing the blood flow to zero. A wide range of diameters exists among capillaries in any given tissue. In skeletal muscle and heart of rats, capillary diameters range from 2 to 8.5 μm [11]. Although the capillaries are larger in frog muscle, a 4-fold range of diameters is again found [12]. Thus, a large range of flow resistance per unit length exists among capillaries. Even with the same driving pressure across them all, a wide range of values of flow per vessel would occur, including some capillaries with diameters too small to allow RBC flow.

Capillaries in skeletal muscle lie, predominantly, parallel to the muscle fibers. Therefore, they must accommodate themselves to continual changes of fiber length. During muscle shortening, the capillaries are forced into a tortuous configuration [11, 13, 14], whereas during muscle extension, longitudinal stretching of capillaries may occur [15]. Both of these processes could exacerbate the heterogeneity of cross section along each capillary, with consequences for RBC flow. In addition, during muscle extension, a reduction of capillary mean diameter is likely to occur. Thus in rat diaphragm, a reduction of mean diameter from 4.75 to 4.1 μm was found, as sarcomere length increased from 2.3 to 2.9 μm [16].

Each capillary path is punctuated by branch points, both diverging and converging, distributed randomly

[Poisson, see ref. 17] along its length. This produces a network structure of many separate capillary segments, the flow parameters changing as blood passes from one segment to the next. The segment lengths form an exponential distribution [17]. The significant differences in magnitude of capillary network parameters measured in hyperemic versus resting muscles [medial gastrocnemius, gracilis, soleus of rat; see ref. 18] indicate that for periods as long as 1–2 min, some capillaries (all muscles, especially soleus) and some arterioles (gracilis, soleus) remain unperfused in resting muscle but are 'recruited' during hyperemia.

The network structure of capillary beds must give rise to a wide range of driving pressures across the constituent segments, extending down to zero in the case of interconnecting channels and with the possibility of flow reversals. Every time a RBC or leukocyte enters a diverging bifurcation and sandbags momentarily over the apex, the flow will be perturbed and detectable 'echoes' may occur throughout the network. At converging bifurcations, an interesting situation often arises [19] when two RBCs, one from each afferent capillary, arrive at the same instant and tend to jam the entrance to the efferent vessel. The minicylindrical diameter for two RBCs is approximately 5 μm as opposed to 2.9 μm for a single RBC, and it may be for this reason that capillaries become larger in diameter towards the venous end of a network. Certainly, the events that occur when RBCs or leukocytes enter a confluence will cause flow perturbations throughout the network, just as do events at diverging bifurcations.

The complexity of a capillary network must lead to an inherent spatial heterogeneity of vascular resistances and thus of flow among vessels, even if the perfusate were a simple Newtonian fluid. However, in that case, the spatial heterogeneity of perfusion would remain constant with time. In contrast, when capillary networks are perfused by blood, we would predict the spatial heterogeneity to be dynamic, due to the two-phase nature of capillary blood flow. As RBCs enter and leave a capillary segment, they alter the resistance to flow within that segment, leading to a redistribution of blood flow and of RBCs between daughter branches at diverging bifurcations.

RBC Flow in Capillary Networks

Based on capillary network morphology, we would expect enormous flow heterogeneity, both spatial and temporal, among the vessel segments which make up any network. In order to quantify this heterogeneity we have

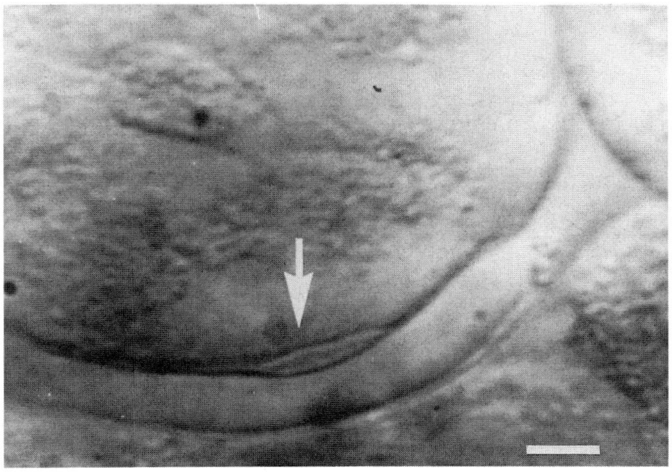

Fig. 3. Intravital videomicroscopic view of capillary running along the border of acinar cells in mouse exocrine pancreas. The nuclear region of an endothelial cell (arrow) bulges into the lumen, narrowing the vessel. Bar = 10 μm. Modified from MacDonald et al. [6].

made continuous (10/s) measurements of RBC velocity [20], lineal density [cells/mm; see ref. 21], and supply rate [cells/s; see ref. 22] in individual capillaries over periods of several minutes, based on computer analysis of recorded video images. Repeated video playback allowed the study of many capillaries 'simultaneously', in the same field of view.

The concept of temporal heterogeneity of RBC supply rate within individual capillaries in resting muscle [23] may be appreciated from figure 4, which shows fluctuations by more than an order of magnitude occurring on a second-to-second basis. When the 6,000 data points accumulated from each capillary over a 10-min period are presented as histograms (fig. 5), both the temporal heterogeneity and the differences of RBC supply rate among capillaries (referred to as 'spatial' heterogeneity) become quite obvious. From the standpoint of functional capillary density, it is particularly striking that capillaries with a very low mean RBC supply rate (many of which are observed in resting muscle) show periods of zero or near-zero flow. In terms of spatial heterogeneity, however, the three capillaries represented in figure 5 came from sartorius muscles of different frogs, and the marked differences in RBC mean supply rate could be due to either the animals, the arterioles, or the capillary network. To distinguish differences among capillaries that are due solely to the capillary network itself, it is therefore necessary to study the temporal and spatial heterogeneity of RBC perfusion in capillary networks that are supplied by a single arteriole [24].

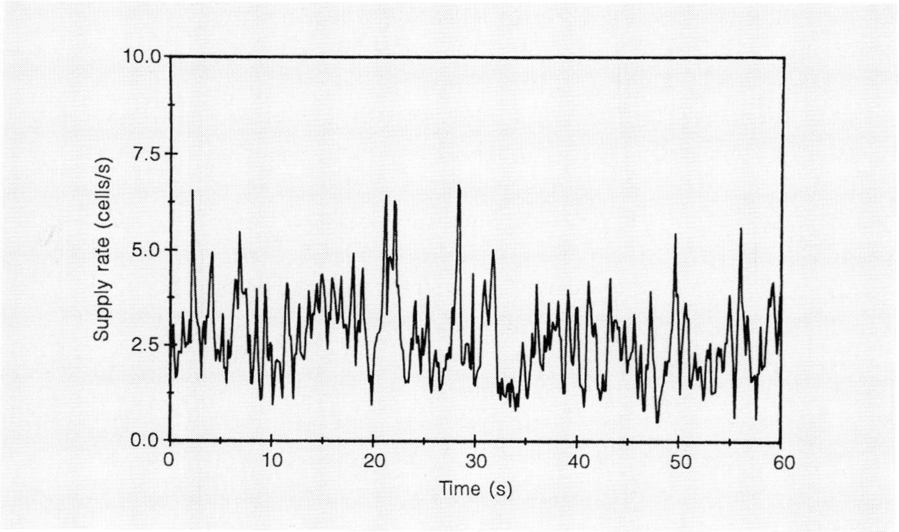

Fig. 4. Temporal heterogeneity of RBC supply rate within a capillary at the surface of rat gracilis muscle. Fluctuations by more than an order magnitude can occur on a second-to-second basis. Modified from Ellis et al. [23].

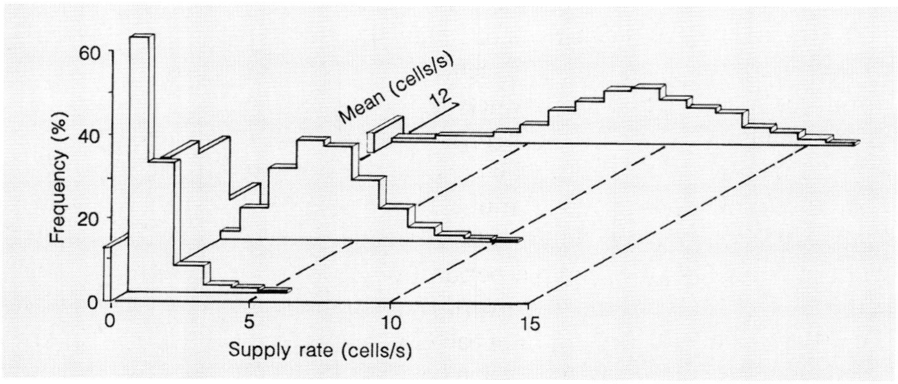

Fig. 5. Histograms of RBC supply rate data for three different capillaries from frog sartorius muscle, over a 10-min period. Each temporal histogram contains 6,000 values. The histogram on the diagonal axis shows the distribution of mean values for all 46 capillaries sampled. Modified from Ellis et al. [23].

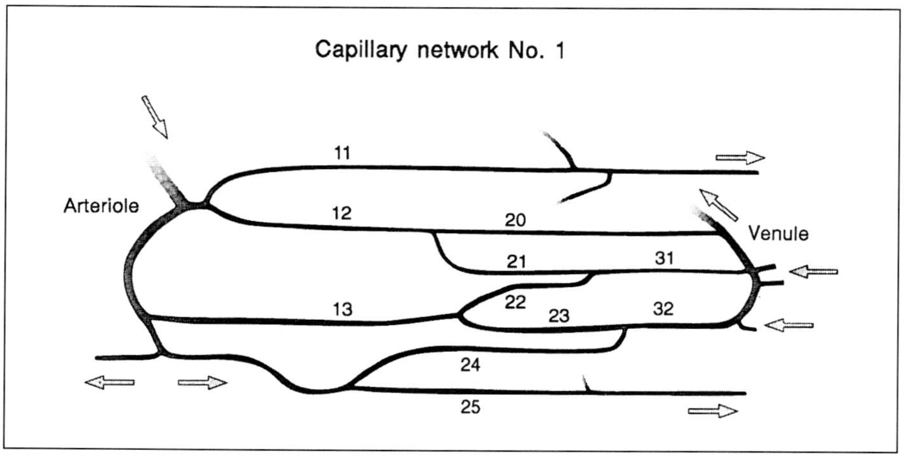

Fig. 6. Schematic of a capillary network from frog sartorius muscle. Direction of flow is indicated by the arrows. Each segment has been identified with a two-digit code, the first digit indicating whether it is a first-, second-, or third-order vessel and the second digit specifying the particular segment within each branching order. From Ellis et al. [24].

The schematic diagram of such a network (fig. 6) identifies the set of numbered capillary segments in which RBC perfusion was measured over the same 10-min interval. (The first digit denotes 1st-, 2nd- or 3rd-order vessels and the second digit specifies the particular segment within each branching order.) For each RBC supply parameter in turn (i.e. velocity, lineal density, supply rate), mean values in each individual segment were computed for each of 60 successive 10-second intervals, each interval corresponding to a new set of RBCs within the network. These data are displayed in the form of a 3-dimensional (3D) plot in figure 7. The shaded face on the lower right of the figure reveals the variation of RBC supply rate with time (bold line) for capillary segment 11, and the successive planes parallel to this, but toward the left, show the variation for segments 12 to 25. The shaded face on the lower left indicates the variation in RBC supply rate among the nine segments during the first 10-second interval. To highlight such differences, at each subsequent time interval, a line has been drawn connecting the values for all capillary segments. 3D plots such as this give a visual impression of both spatial and temporal heterogeneity of RBC perfusion in capillary networks supplied by a single arteriole. 'Mountain ranges' versus 'valleys' reveal persistent differences between capillaries (compare segments 20 and 21, or 24 and 25). The results leave no doubt that enormous flow heterogeneity, both spatial and temporal, exists among the vessel segments of a capillary network. Moreover, the origin of this heterogeneity is not only the arteriolar supply but the capillary network itself.

The spatial and temporal heterogeneity observed in such 3D plots may be quantified by computing values of the mean and SD for each flow parameter among capillaries at each successive time interval (spatial), and for each capillary over the entire sample period (temporal). The arteriolar RBC supply to the network can be computed from the sum of the supply rates in each first-order capillary segment. In this way, the overall heterogeneity of perfusion may be resolved into two components, spatial and temporal, both being expressed in terms of coefficients of variation (CV%: SD/mean × 100). Some interesting further concepts then emerge.

The first concept is that the spatial heterogeneity of RBC flow within capillary networks is dynamic in nature. This is illustrated by figure 8, in which the spatial CV% for 10-second mean values of capillary RBC velocity, in the network presented earlier (fig. 6), ranged from < 30 to > 55% over a 10-min period. The dashed line in figure 8 shows the variation in the arteriolar RBC supply rate to the network during this same period of time, and it is clear that an inverse relationship exists between the peaks and valleys of the two sets of data. It has been reported from a study on hemodilution [25] that the RBC flow distribution within the mesenteric capillary bed depends on the hematocrit of the inflowing blood. This indicates that blood rheology plays an important role in determining capillary flow distribution. The same thing should occur on a dynamic basis, and figure 8 suggests that this may be the case in resting muscle. Clear evidence that this is so emerges when the spatial CV values for capillary 10-second mean RBC velocity are plotted against the corresponding values of arteriolar RBC supply rate (fig. 9). Our recent studies [24] demonstrate unequivocally that there are dynamic redistributions of RBC flow within the network and that the greater the arteriolar RBC supply to a network, the more homogeneous the capillary perfusion.

The second concept is that the temporal heterogeneity of RBC flow in a capillary may be several-fold higher than

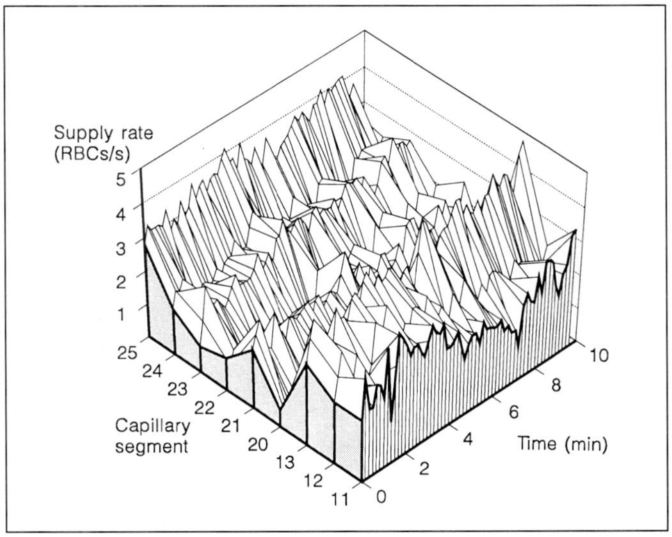

Fig. 7. 3D plot of RBC supply rate vs. capillary segment ID vs. time, for the capillary network shown in figure 6. ID refers to the two-digit code identifying each capillary segment. Modified from Ellis et al. [24].

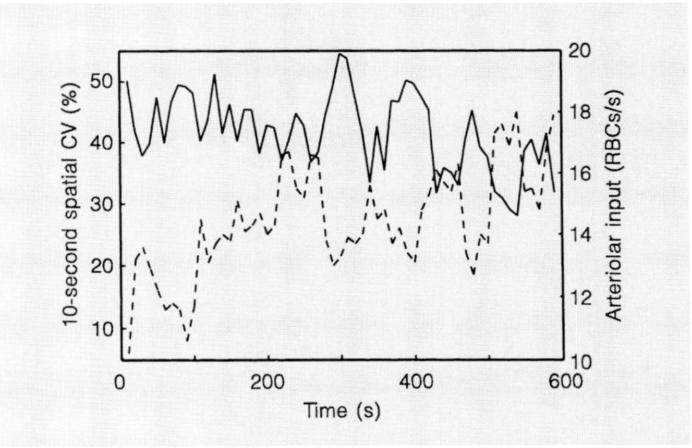

Fig. 8. Variation in the spatial heterogeneity of capillary RBC velocity with time (—— = 10-second spatial CV) for the network shown in figure 6. The estimated arteriolar input RBC supply rate is also plotted (– – –). Note the inverse relationship between peaks and valleys of the two sets of data.

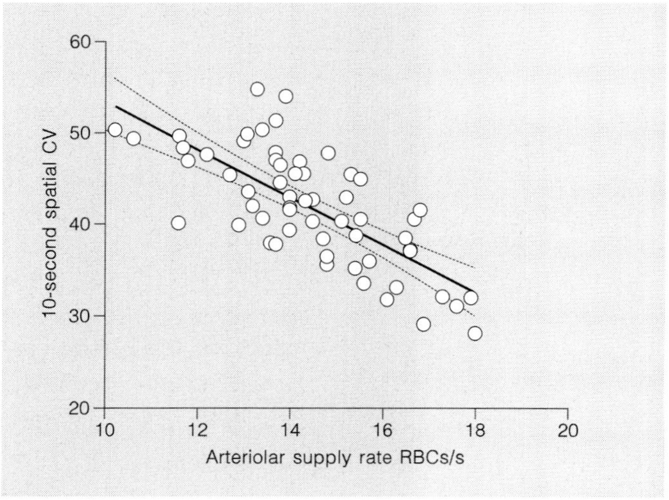

9

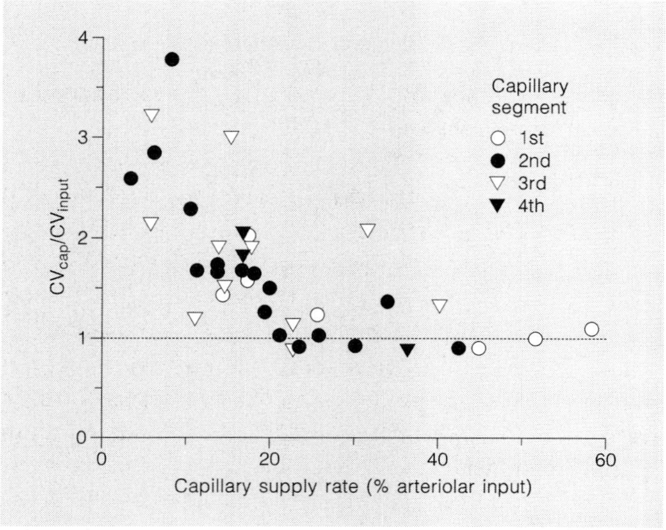

10

Fig. 9. Variations in the spatial heterogeneity of capillary RBC velocity (10-second spatial CV) for the network shown in figure 6, as a scatter plot vs. the estimated arteriolar RBC supply rate. —— = The least-squares regression line; ····· = 95% confidence intervals. Modified from Ellis et al. [24].

Fig. 10. Relative temporal heterogeneity of capillary supply rate (CV_{cap}/CV_{input}, where cap is capillary RBC supply, and input is arteriolar input) vs. capillary RBC supply rate expressed as a percentage of the arteriolar input supply rate. The data have been pooled from five networks. The order of the capillary segment from which the data were obtained is indicated by the different symbols shown in the legend. From Ellis et al. [24].

in the supplying arteriole, depending on how much of the total inflow the vessel receives. This may be seen from figure 10, which shows that temporal redistributions of RBC flow among capillaries were particularly evident with vessels carying less than 20% of the arteriolar input. Such vessels showed temporal CV values up to 4-fold that

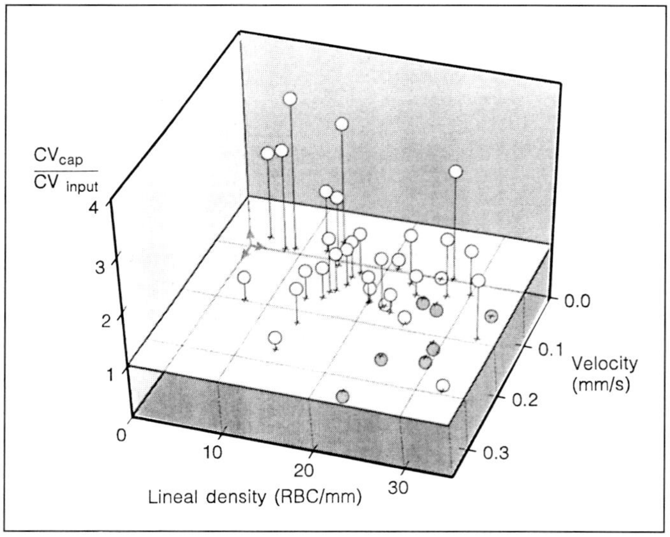

Fig. 11. 3D plot of the relative temporal heterogeneity of supply rate (CV_{cap}/CV_{input}, where cap is capillary supply, and input is arteriolar input) vs. velocity vs. lineal density. The origin of the plot is shown by the arrows in the lower back corner of the graph. The plane at $CV_{cap}/CV_{input} = 1.0$ indicates the level at which the temporal heterogeneity of the capillary equals that of the input. The distance between a data point and this plane is indicated by the thin vertical line. The location of the point in the velocity versus lineal density plane is shown by a small + drawn in perspective. All values above the plane are white; all values below the plane are shaded gray. From Ellis et al. [24].

of the arteriolar supply, regardless of their segment branching order within the network. When these same CV ratios are considered in relation to the corresponding values of capillary RBC velocity and lineal density (fig. 11), it becomes clear that vessels with the highest relative temporal heterogeneity of perfusion were characterized by both low velocity and low lineal density of RBCs. In general, however, the relative heterogeneity depended more strongly on RBC velocity than on the number of RBCs per unit length of capillary.

Network Perfusion Concepts Relevant to Functional Capillary Density

The title of this symposium gives recognition to the fact that there are passive as well as active determinants of functional capillary density. Arising from capillary network morphology and the rheological events that occur when RBCs pass through a network, considerable heterogeneity of perfusion is to be expected at the capillary level. Our studies have quantified this heterogeneity and the results permit a number of conclusions to be drawn that are important for an understanding of passive determinants of functional capillary density.

First of all, even with a high arteriolar RBC supply, persistent differences in perfusion among capillaries remain, due to network geometry. The mean spatial CV value for capillary RBC supply in networks fed by a single arteriole was 47%, more than two-thirds of the value of 66% obtained when interarteriolar and animal-to-animal variations were included. This indicates that the capillary network itself is the primary source of the heterogeneity of RBC perfusion. Second, within the capillary network, RBC flow continuously redistributes among capillaries. This is shown by a 3-fold variation with time in the 10-second spatial CV value for RBC velocity and lineal density, and 2-fold variation in the corresponding value for RBC supply rate.

A third conclusion is that the spatial heterogeneity of capillary RBC flow increases substantially as the arteriolar input to the network falls. This suggests that the fractional distribution of RBCs at capillary bifurcations depends not only on the flow distribution [26] but also on the magnitude of the RBC supply in the parent vessel. During periods of low RBC input to the network, RBCs would be found primarily in preferential paths, whereas during high RBC input, the distribution would be more uniform amongst all flow paths. In other words, during low-flow states, the network will fail to distribute blood properly among its constituent capillaries. As the inflow to the network rises, more vessels will be 'recruited' to carry flow.

A fourth conclusion is that the capillaries with the lowest flow exhibit the highest temporal heterogeneity of perfusion, which means that these vessels are the most easily 'recruited' or blocked. These capillaries had the lowest RBC velocities, indicating that the driving pressure relative to hemodynamic resistance across these segments was small. Therefore, these vessels would be the most susceptible to plugging by leukocytes or stiffened RBCs at low flow rates. If such capillary segments are 'lost' as far as perfusion is concerned, then the ability of the network to reduce its heterogeneity and increase its efficiency for exchange will be impaired, and in fact the heterogeneity will shift towards higher values. The existence in resting muscle of a proportion of capillaries having zero or near-zero flow has also been demonstrated [18] by percutaneous intracardiac injection of a small bolus of colloidal carbon suspension.

Our conclusion is that whereas the arterior network *actively* controls the input of blood to capillary networks, it is the capillary network geometry and the rheological properties of blood in these networks that determine, *passively,* the flow distribution among capillary segments and which segments will lose their flow when the arteriolar inflow is reduced. A similar conclusion was reached by Lindbom and Arfors [27], who measured RBC velocities in capillaries originating from a single terminal arteriole in vasodilated tenuissimus muscle, following stepwise reductions in hindlimb perfusion pressure. They found that the higher the velocity in a capillary during perfusion at 65 mm Hg, the lower the perfusion pressure at which flow stasis developed. As the pressure was progressively reduced below 30 mm Hg, more and more vessels showed stasis, until at 15 mm Hg only 2 out of 9 vessels remained perfused. These results demonstrate that the density of perfused capillaries is a function of the pressure gradient across the network.

Implications for Microvascular Oxygen Exchange in Skeletal Muscle

Increasing the homogeneity of RBC perfusion in capillary networks is expected, intuitively, to lead to an increased efficiency of O_2 exchange between blood and tissue. In resting muscle, we have shown that there is, on average, a high spatial heterogeneity of perfusion. Furthermore, this spatial heterogeneity is highly variable with time. These findings lead inevitably to the conclusion that resting muscle is perfectly able to tolerate a wide range of spatial heterogeneity of RBC perfusion. It has recently been reported [28] that in resting muscle, O_2 exchange occurs among capillaries and between arterioles and capillaries. Thus, the reason why such a high perfusion heterogeneity can be tolerated in resting muscle may be that it is the integrated supply of a group of capillaries which determines tissue oxygenation, not the supply in each capillary independent of its neighbors.

In exercising muscle, there is a greatly increased tissue O_2 demand, as a result of which the degree of diffusive exchange among microvessels will decrease and the spatial heterogeneity of capillary perfusion will become important. The level of heterogeneity tolerated at rest may now result in local regions of ischemia. However, as indicated above, a passive rheological mechanism is already in place to reduce perfusion heterogeneity significantly as the RBC supply rate increases in response to increased O_2 demand. Nevertheless, the heterogeneity cannot be abolished entirely. There is a further passive mechanism which may contribute to improved tissue oxygenation. This is the phenomenon of capillary tortuosity which develops as a consequence of muscle shortening [11]. A network of tortuous capillaries may lead to a relatively uniform O_2 source around the periphery of muscle fibers, providing a more efficient geometry for exchange than that of a central O_2 source [29, 30].

In resting and also in exercising skeletal muscle, it is clear that active and passive elements are interwoven in determining functional capillary density and O_2 transport to tissue.

Acknowledgement

Supported by separate grants to A.C.G. and C.G.E. from the Heart and Stroke Foundation of Ontario. C.G.E. is a Career Investigator of the Heart and Stroke Foundation.

References

1 Plyley MJ: The Organization of the Capillary Network in Skeletal Muscle; PhD thesis University of Western Ontario, 1977.
2 Groom AC, Ellis CG, Wrigley S, Potter RF: Architecture and flow patterns in capillary networks of skeletal muscle in frog and rat; in Popel AS, Johnson PC (eds): Microvascular Networks: Experimental and Theoretical Studies. Basel, Karger, 1986, pp 61–76.
3 McCuskey RS, Chapman TM: Microscopy of the living pancreas in situ. Am J Anat 1969; 126:395–408.
4 Ragan DMS, Schmidt EE, MacDonald IC, Groom AC: Spontaneous cyclic contractions of the capillary wall in vivo, impeding red cell flow: A quantitative analysis. Evidence for endothelial contractility. Microvasc Res 1988;36: 13–30.
5 Aharinejad S, MacDonald IC, Schmidt EE, Böck P, Hagen D, Groom AC: Scanning and transmission electron microscopy and high resolution intravital videomicroscopy of capillaries in the mouse exocrine pancreas, with special emphasis on endothelial cells. Anat Rec 1993;237:163–177.
6 MacDonald IC, Aharinejad S, Schmidt EE, Groom AC: Luminal constrictions due to endothelial cells in capillaries of mouse exocrine pancreas. Microvasc Res 1995;49:64–77.
7 Ellis CG, Tyml K, Burgess W: Quantification of red cell movement in microvessels: A new application of interactive computer graphics. Microvasc Res 1987;33:428–432.
8 Ellis CG, Tyml K, Strang BK: Variation in axial velocity profile of red cells passing through a single capillary. Adv Exp Med Biol 1989;248:543–550.
9 Kiani MF, Cokelet GR, Sarelius IH: Effect of diameter variability along a microvessel segment on pressure drop. Microvasc Res 1993; 45:219–232.
10 Secomb TW: Flow dependent rheological properties of blood in capillaries. Microvasc Res 1987;34:46–58.
11 Potter RF, Groom AC: Capillary diameter and geometry in cardiac and skeletal muscle studied by means of corrosion casts. Microvasc Res 1983;25:68–84.
12 Safranyos RGA, Ellis CG, Tyml K, Groom AC: Heterogeneity of capillary diameters in skeletal muscle of the frog. Microvasc Res 1983;26: 151–156.
13 Mathieu-Costello O: Capillary tortuosity and degree of contraction or extension of skeletal muscle. Microvasc Res 1987;33:98–117.
14 Mathieu-Costello O, Potter RF, Ellis CG, Groom AC: Capillary configuration and fiber shortening in muscles of the rat hindlimb: Correlation between corrosion casts and stereological measurements. Microvasc Res 1988;36:40–55.
15 Ellis CG, Mathieu-Costello O, Potter RF, MacDonald IC, Groom AC: Effect of sarcomere length on total capillary length in skeletal muscle: In vivo evidence for longitudinal stretching of capillaries. Microvasc Res 1990;40:63–72.
16 Poole DC, Mathieu-Costello O: Capillary and fiber geometry in rat diaphragm perfusion fixed in situ at different sarcomere lengths. J Appl Physiol 1992;73:151–159.
17 Plyley MJ, Sutherland GJ, Groom AC: Geometry of the capillary network in skeletal muscle. Microvasc Res 1976;11:161–173.
18 Potter RF, Houghton S, Groom AC: Capillary lengths and anastomoses in rat hindlimb muscles, studies by Aquablak perfusion during rest versus exercise. Adv Exp Med Biol 1989;248: 313–322.
19 Wells SM, Potter RF, Sainani DR, Ellis CG: Red blood cell flow at converging capillary bifurcations (abstract M117). FASEB J 1992;6: A2088.
20 Tyml K, Sherebrin MH: A method for on-line measurements of red cell velocity in microvessels using computerized frame-by-frame analysis of television images. Microvasc Res 1980; 20:1–8.
21 Ellis CG, Fraser S, Hamilton G, Groom AC: Measurement of the lineal density of red blood cells in capillaries in vivo, using a computerized frame-by-frame analysis of video images. Microvasc Res 1984;27:1–13.
22 Ellis CG, Tyml K, Groom AC: Computer-assisted analysis of video images: A new tool for microvascular measurement; in Baker CH, Nastuk WL (eds): Microcirculatory Technology. New York, Academic Press, 1986, pp 229–244.
23 Ellis CG, Wrigley SM, Potter RF, Groom AC: Temporal distributions of red cell supply rate to individual capillaries of resting skeletal muscle in frog and rat. Int J Microcirc Clin Exp 1990;9:67–84.
24 Ellis CG, Wrigley SM, Groom AC: Heterogeneity of red cell perfusion in capillary networks supplied by a single arteriole, in resting skeletal muscle. Circ Res 1994;75:357–368.
25 Pries AR, Fritzsche A, Ley K, Gaehtgens P: Redistribution of red blood cell flow in microcirculatory networks by hemodilution. Circ Res 1992;70:1113–1121.
26 Pries AR, Ley K, Claasen M, Gaehtgens P: Red cell distribution at microvascular bifurcations. Microvasc Res 1989;38:81–101.
27 Lindbom L, Arfors KE: Mechanisms and site of control for variation in the number of perfused capillaries in skeletal muscle. Int J Microcirc Clin Exp 1985;4:19–30.
28 Ellsworth ML, Ellis CG, Popel AS, Pittman RN: Role of microvessels in oxygen supply to tissue. News Physiol Sci 1994;9:119–123.
29 Ellis CG, Potter RF, Groom AC: The Krogh cylinder geometry is not appropriate for modelling O_2 transport in contracted skeletal muscle. Adv Med Biol 1983;159:253–268.
30 Groom AC, Ellis CG, Potter RF: Microvascular architecture and red cell perfusion in skeletal muscle: Changes during shortening and possible improvement in oxygen transport to tissue; in Messmer K, Hammersen F (eds): Skeletal Muscle Microcirculation. Prog Appl Microcirc. Basel, Karger, 1984, vol 5, pp 64–83.

Int J Microcirc 1995;15:231–237

O. Mathieu-Costello[a]
L. H. Manciet[b]
K. Tyml[c]

[a] Department of Medicine, University of California, San Diego, La Jolla, Calif.,
[b] Department of Surgery, University of Arizona Health Sciences Center, Tucson, Ariz., USA; and
[c] Department of Medical Biophysics, University of Western Ontario, and the Robarts Research Institute, London, Ontario, Canada

Capillary Ultrastructure and Functional Capillary Density

Key Words
Edema
Perfusion
Red blood cell velocity
Hyperemic response
Disuse
Aging
Ischemia

Abstract
We briefly summarize our findings on alterations in capillary structure in skeletal muscle and heart in response to up to 30 min of ischemia. In frog sartorius muscle, reactive hyperemia was absent in atrophy. Increased spatial heterogeneity of red cell velocity in individual capillaries was observed, as were increases in the percentage of capillaries with damaged endothelium and white cell volume density in capillaries. Examination of the effect of aging on the response of the vascular bed to 30 min ischemia in extensor digitorum longus muscle of Fisher 344 rats suggested that the lack of postischemic hyperemia and structural alterations in frog muscle were related to disuse rather than aging per se. However, the specific study of disuse in rat extensor digitorum longus muscle after chronic application of tetrodotoxin revealed both capillary damage and a postischemic hyperemic response. It suggested an effect of the degree of tissue deterioration on the hyperemic response after short-term disuse in rat muscle, compared to longer-term atrophy in frog. Morphometric data in isolated rabbit heart suggested a link between microvascular compression as a result of tissue edema and decreased perfusion after 30 min total ischemia.

A number of factors, structural and functional, can affect muscle functional capillary density. Ultrastructural alterations in endothelial morphology including cell swelling, changes in capillary diameter or shape, and cell trapping in the vasculature can modify the distribution of perfused vessels, at a given level of total blood flow. Functional changes, not necessarily discernable by electron microscopy, can also profoundly influence the density of perfused capillaries. Endothelial cells can become more or less sticky, or the transmission of signals from the capillary endothelium to the arterial network can be altered, or changes at the level of venules, especially in conditions of low flow can modify red cell flux into the capillaries. Several aspects of capillary morphology, tissue perfusion and blood cell rheology are discussed throughout this issue. In this paper, we focus on capillary ultrastructure and the relationship(s) between alterations at this level and capillary perfusion.

Capillary Damage after Ischemia

There have been a number of studies documenting capillary damage in muscle after severe ischemia. In the heart, Armiger and Gavin [1] found increasing endothelial cell swelling and degeneration after 10–60 min coro-

Odile Mathieu-Costello, PhD
University of California, San Diego
School of Medicine, Section of Physiology
9500 Gilman Drive Dept. 0623
La Jolla, CA 92093-0623 (USA)

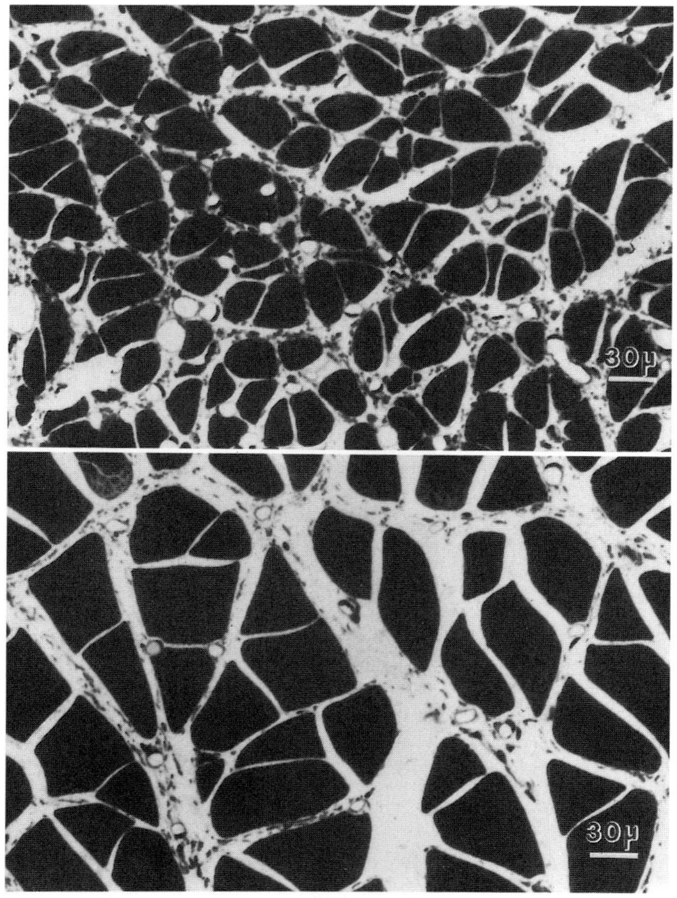

a

b

Fig. 1. Light micrographs of portions of muscle bundles in transverse section of frog sartorius muscle, showing the large decrease in fiber size in atrophied muscle. Fiber mean cross-sectional area (group average) was 568 ± 36 and 1,935 ± 408 μm^2 in atrophied (**a**) (n = 4) and control (**b**) (n = 5) muscles, respectively. From Tyml et al. [4].

nary artery occlusion. Characteristic ultrastructural features of damaged endothelial cells were the presence of cytoplasmic projections into the capillary lumen, membrane-bound profiles, swollen organelles and lipid droplets. However, not all cells were affected to the same extent, adjacent cells showing large differences in their degree of swelling even after 60 min of ischemia, and endothelial cell junctions were preserved [1]. In skeletal muscle, Strock and Majno [2] showed that after 2.5 h of complete ischemia, morphological alterations of the capillary bed were relatively mild; they were focal in nature and widenings between endothelial cells were rare. Morphological alterations of the capillary endothelium included organelle swelling and projection of membranous structures into the capillary lumen. Gidlöf et al. [3] reported similar changes, and a localized endothelial swelling, i.e. alterations in endothelial cells lying next to others ultrastructurally intact in human quadriceps femoris muscle after 90–180 min total ischemia. The duration of ischemia to produce perfusion impairment, i.e. to prevent the expected reactive hyperemia in mammalian skeletal muscle is about 2–3 h, compared to 10–15 min in brain, and 30–60 min in myocardium [3]. In this paper, we summarize studies where we examined (1) endothelial ultrastructure (electron microscopy) and microvascular response (intravital microscopy) to a shorter period of ischemia (30 min) in skeletal muscle [4-6] and microvascular compression (light microscopy and morphometry) in the heart after 5 and 30 min global ischemia [7].

Capillary Ultrastructure and Microvascular Response to Ischemia in Skeletal Muscle

Three series of experiments were conducted where endothelial ultrastructure and microvascular response to 30 min ischemia were examined in three different conditions: muscle atrophy, aging and disuse. Intravital measurements of microvascular function were carried out using methods described by Tyml and Budreau [8, 9], and then the tissue was fixed by superfusion with glutaraldehyde (GA) fixative (6.25% GA in 0.1 *M* sodium cacodylate buffer) in situ for 30 min and processed for electron microscopy as previously described [10].

The effect of muscle atrophy was studied in frog sartorius muscle [4]. Frogs had been kept in captivity for about a year. Body weight was reduced by 50%, and sartorius muscle weight was about 28% that of controls. The dramatic reduction in fiber size in the atrophied muscle is illustrated in figure 1. Capillary anatomical density was much greater in atrophied [892 ± 222 (SD) capillaries/fiber mm^2 cross-sectional area] compared to normal muscle (282 ± 29 capillaries/mm^2). This increased capillary density was entirely due to the difference in fiber size. There was no alteration in capillary-to-fiber ratio with muscle atrophy.

After 30 min complete ischemia induced by compression of a small supplying artery, the hyperemic response seen in the controls did not occur in atrophied muscle (fig. 2a). This was due to a large heterogeneity in the response of the capillary bed in atrophied muscle. Out of 24 randomly chosen capillaries, approximately the same number of vessels showed an increase, a decrease or no change in red cell velocity in response to the ischemia, whereas the majority of capillaries showed an increased flow in normal muscle (fig. 2b). Figure 2c shows that the

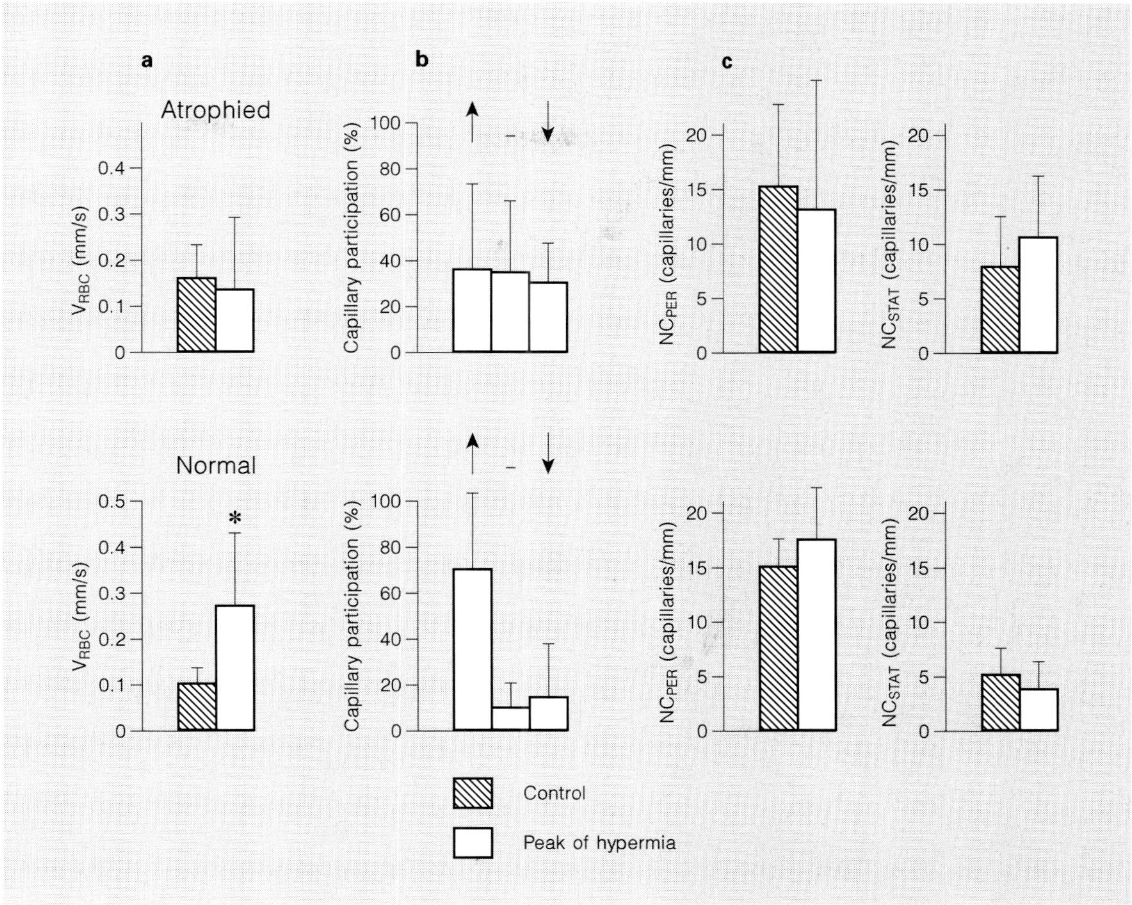

Fig. 2. Functional response of the capillary bed of frog muscle to ischemia. Error bars = SD. Adapted from Tyml et al. [4]. **a** Microvascular response to 30 min arterial occlusion in atrophied (n = 8) and normal (n = 7) frog sartorius muscles. V_{RBC} = Red cell velocity. * $p < 0.05$ compared to control. **b** Capillary participation represented as the percentage of capillaries showing increase (↑), no change (–) or decrease (↓) in red cell velocity compared to preocclusion values. **c** Number of capillaries with moving red cells (NC_{PER}) and with stationary red cells (NC_{STAT}) in atrophied (n = 8) and normal (n = 7) frog sartorius muscle.

number of capillaries with moving red cells and those with stationary cells were not significantly different between the two groups, but there was an increased spatial heterogeneity in the response of the capillary bed in the atrophied muscles. It also illustrates the coarser description of vascular response when one considers vascular function in terms of capillaries perfused or not (fig. 2c) instead of rates of velocity within perfused capillaries (fig. 2a). The quantification of capillary damage, identified by a thickened endothelium and the presence of increased capillary folding and projections into the lumen compared to normal ultrastructure (fig. 3) revealed a 3-fold increase in the percentage of capillaries with damaged endothelium in atrophied muscle (33.5 ± 1.6%) compared to normal muscle (12.6 ± 0.9%). This increase was accompanied by an increased volume density of white cells per volume of capillary (atrophied, 2.0 ± 0.1; normal 0.8 ± 0.0%).

The impaired vascular function observed in the atrophied frog muscle could be attributed to either aging or disuse, since both occurred in this experimental model. The two following studies were carried out to possibly dissociate the effect of aging from that of disuse. They were made possible by the development of a method to examine the microvasculature of the rat hindlimb by intravital microscopy [9].

The effect of aging on the response of the vascular bed to 30 min ischemia and its relation to capillary structure

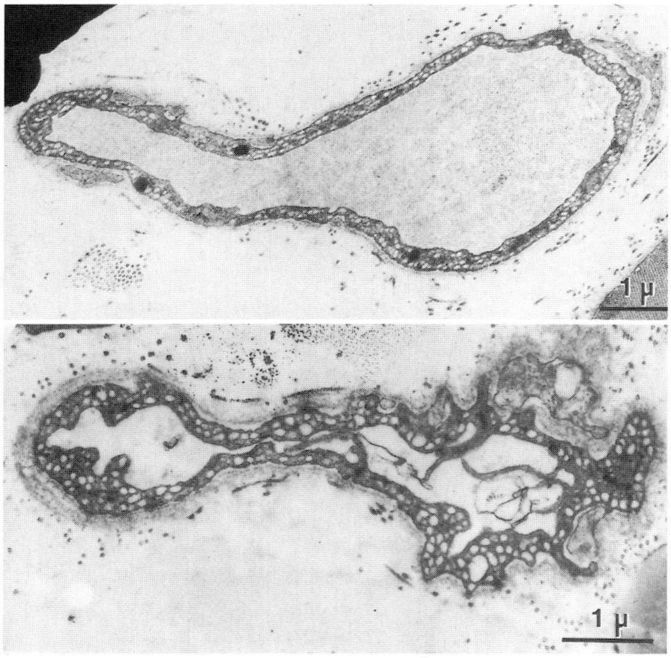

a

b

Fig. 3. Examples of capillary profiles with normal endothelial ultrastructure (**a**) compared to damaged endothelium (**b**), in frog sartorius muscle. From Tyml et al. [4].

were studied in rat extensor digitorum longus (EDL) [5]. In old (28 months) Fisher 344 rats, there was an increase in the absolute spread of red blood cell (RBC) velocities in individual capillaries compared to mid-aged (12 months) rats (fig. 4a). However, the coefficient of variation, i.e. the spread of RBC velocities in individual capillaries relative to the mean was approximately the same (90%), indicating that there was no change in the spatial heterogeneity in RBC velocities in the capillary network with aging. After 30 min complete ischemia produced by a tourniquet around the knee, a hyperemic response was also seen in old rats, but it was slower to return to preischemic RBC velocity values than in mid-aged rat (fig. 4b). Wet/dry weight ratios, measured in the tibialis anterior, revealed no sign of edema after the 30-min ischemia in either group, and practically no capillary damage was found. Out of 91 and 86 capillaries sampled in 5 muscles in each group, 2 and 1 vessels showed abnormal ultrastructure in the old and mid-aged group, respectively. Thus, the data suggested that the lack of hyperemic response and the structural alterations found in the frog muscles could be related to disuse rather than aging per se.

The effect of disuse on capillary ultrastructure and the functional response of the capillary bed to ischemia were examined in the EDL of mid-aged (12 months) Fisher 344 rats after 2 weeks neural application of tetrodotoxin (TTX) on the sciatic nerve [6]. This produced a decrease in muscle weight of about 40%, and an approximately 50% decrease in fiber cross-sectional area, from 1,585 ± 168 μm^2 in normal muscles (5 animals) to 767 ± 62 μm^2 in disused muscles (n = 4); both values at 2.1 μm sarcomere length. However, the absolute anatomical number of capillaries was maintained, as observed in the previous study of frog sartorius muscle. On the other hand, intravital microscopy analysis showed that the number of perfused capillaries, i.e. those with moving red cells, significantly increased by about 35% in disused muscles, whereas the density of capillaries with stationary red cells was unaltered (fig. 5a). This contrasts with the study of frog muscle, where neither the number of perfused capillaries, nor of capillaries with stationary cells was altered in response to ischemia. As seen in rat EDL muscle with aging (fig. 4a), the absolute spread of red cell velocities was increased with disuse, but the coefficient of variation relative to the mean was similar, indicating that spatial heterogeneity was unchanged. After 30 min complete ischemia via a tourniquet around the knee, there was a substantial hyperemic response in disused muscle, and return to preischemic levels 20 min after ischemia (fig. 5b). The examination of capillary ultrastructure (29–30 capillaries chosen by systematic random sampling in each of 4 TTX-treated muscles) revealed a greater incidence of capillary damage in disused muscles (11% compared to 1% in controls). Tissue edema was also evidenced by a significant increase in tibialis anterior wet/dry weight ratio. Thus, contrary to the frog sartorius muscle, disused rat EDL showed both capillary damage *and* a hyperemic response to short-term ischemia. The different response may be due to a difference in the degree of tissue deterioration between the two experimental models. The atrophy in rat muscle was short term (2 weeks), while it was longer (1 year) in the frog. In the TTX-treated rat muscle, both muscle atrophy (40%) and capillary damage (11%) were lower than in frog sartorius (64 and 33%, respectively). Capillary perfusion was maintained in rat muscle, whereas only 60% of capillaries were perfused in frog sartorius muscle with atrophy. There is evidence that the degree of hyperemia is inversely related to the degree of capillary damage. This could explain the absence of hyperemic response in frog muscle, while it was present after the disuse protocol used in rat EDL [6].

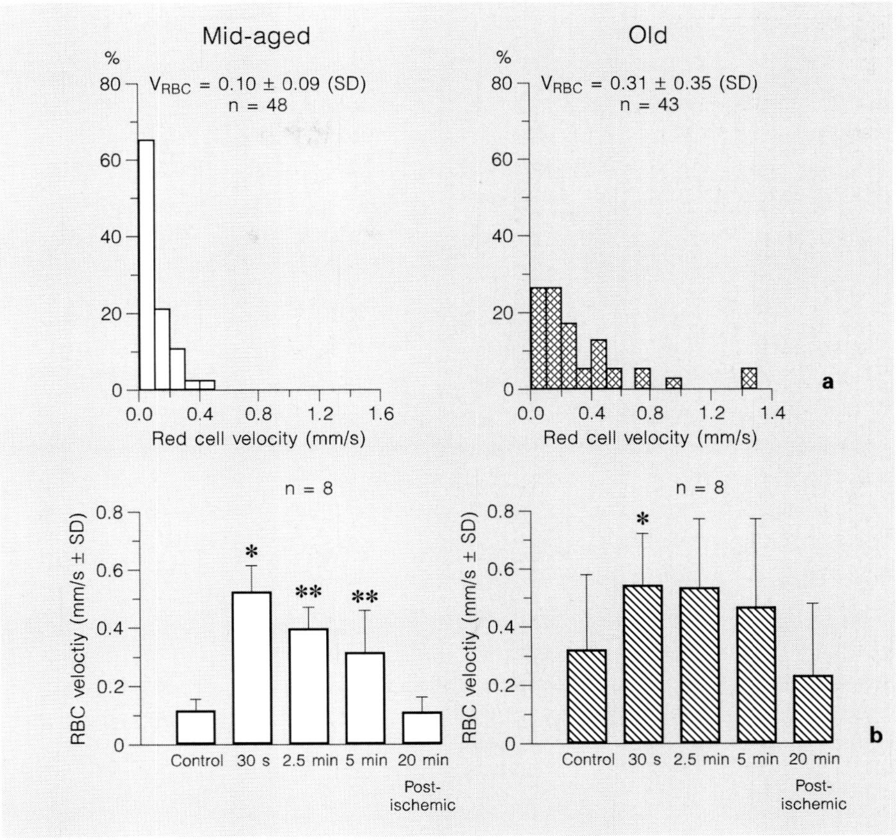

Fig. 4. Effect of aging of the microvascular response in rat muscle. Adapted from Tyml et al. [5]. **a** Distribution of red cell velocities in 48 and 43 capillaries measured within a 0.06-mm^3 sampling volume in one resting EDL muscle from one mid-aged and one old rat. **b** Velocity response to 30 min complete ischemia in EDL muscles of mid-aged and old rats (n = 8 in each group). * = Significantly greater ($p < 0.05$) than control resting value; ** = significantly lower than at 30 s.

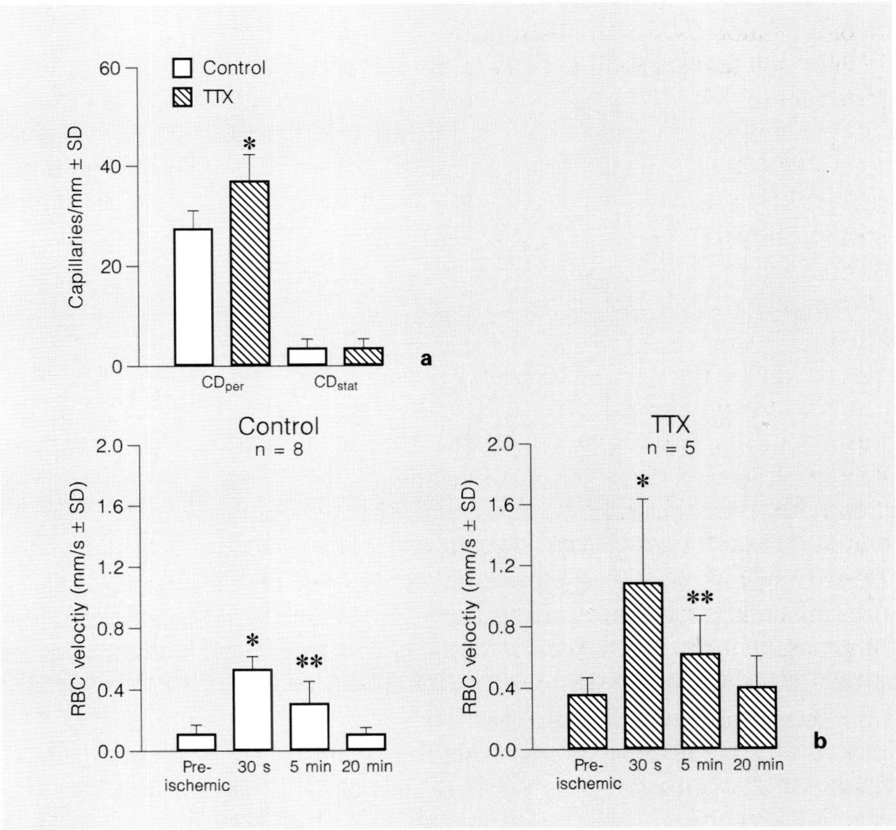

Fig. 5. Effect of disuse on microvascular response in rat muscle. Adapted from Tyml et al. [6]. **a** Density of capillaries with moving red cells (CD_{per}) and stationary red cells (CD_{stat}) in rat extensor digitorum longus following 2 weeks application of TTX on the sciatic nerve (n = 5) and in controls (n = 8). * = Significantly greater ($p < 0.05$) than control. **b** RBC velocity response to 30 min complete ischemia in the same muscle. * = Significantly greater than preischemic value; ** = significantly lower than at 30 s.

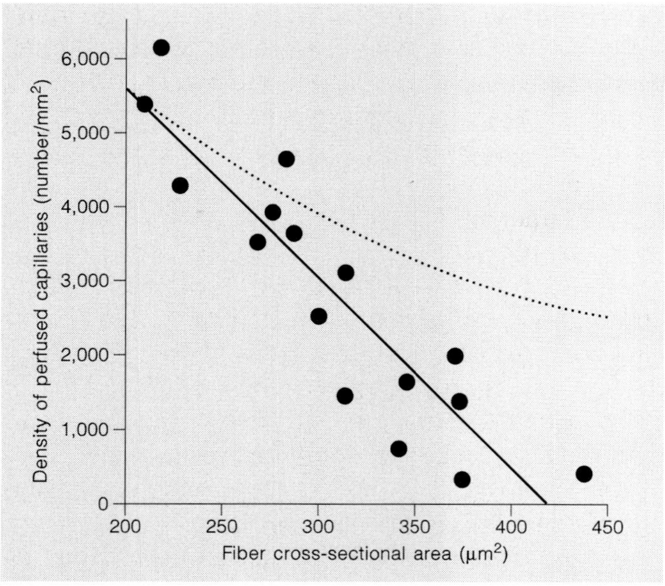

Fig. 6. Relationship between the density of perfused capillaries and fiber cross-sectional area in rabbit heart (n = 16) after 5 and 30 min global ischemia. The measured decrease in capillary density (——; r = 0.92) is greater than that expected from the sole increase in fiber size (----), suggesting that obstruction to flow accompanied the tissue edema (see text). Adapted from Manciet et al. [7].

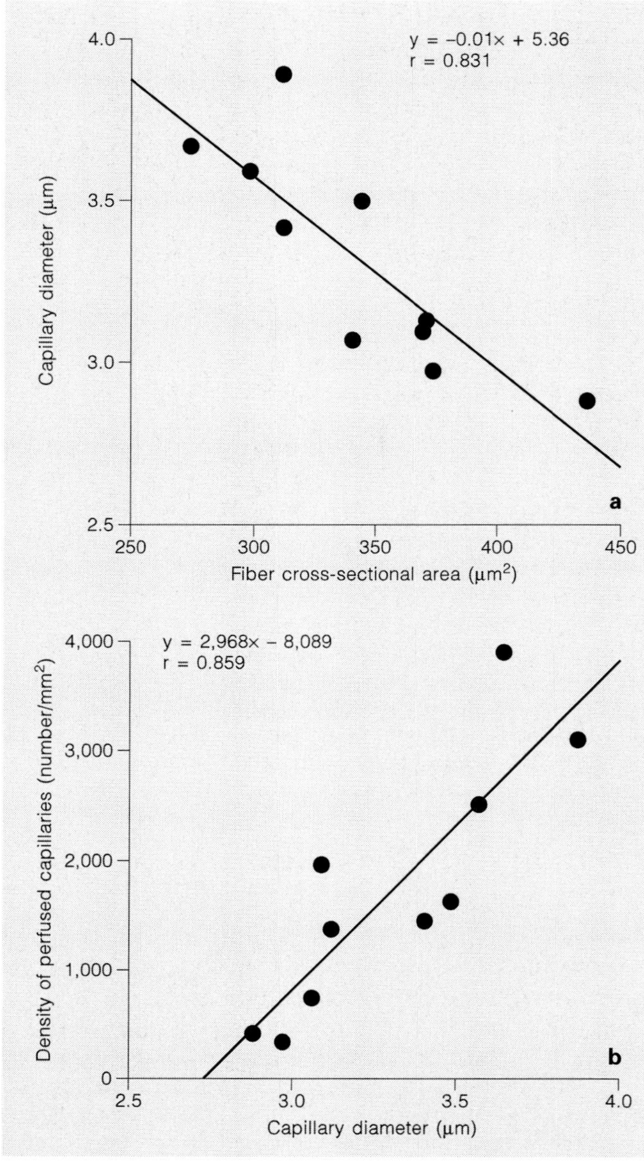

Fig. 7. Inverse relationship between capillary diameter and fiber cross-sectional area (**a**), and correlation between the density of perfused capillaries and decreased capillary diameter (**b**) after 30 min global ischemia in rabbit heart. Adapted from Manciet et al. [7].

Tissue Edema, Capillary Size and Number of Perfused Capillaries in the Myocardium after Ischemia

In this study [7], 5 and 30 min of total ischemia in isolated rabbit heart were followed by perfusion with india ink to identify the density of perfused capillaries, and then fixation with GA solution for microscopic analysis and morphometry. After 30 min ischemia, the density of perfused capillaries in subepicardium and subendocardium regions sampled in the central area of the left ventricular free wall were reduced to less than 50% compared to 5 min ischemia. Fiber cross-sectional area, normalized to sarcomere length, increased significantly (subendocardium: 19%, subepicardium: 40%), indicative of tissue edema. However, the density of perfused capillaries decreased more than expected from the increase in fiber size, indicating that there was obstruction to flow after 30 min ischemia (fig. 6). Capillary diameter was inversely related to fiber cross-sectional area (r = 0.83), and the density of perfused capillaries was also strongly correlated (r = 0.86) with capillary diameter (fig. 7). This suggested a link between microvascular compression as a result of tissue edema and the decreased perfusion after 30 min ischemia. An important additional factor in microvascular compression is interstitial edema. Unfortunately, this quantity is difficult to assess in histological sections. The interstitial space is unreliably preserved during tissue preparation [11]. This is illustrated in figure 8 which shows large differences in interfiber spacing between two adjacent portions of muscle bundles in the same section, i.e. adjacent tissue subjected to rigorously identical preparative steps during processing for electron microscopy.

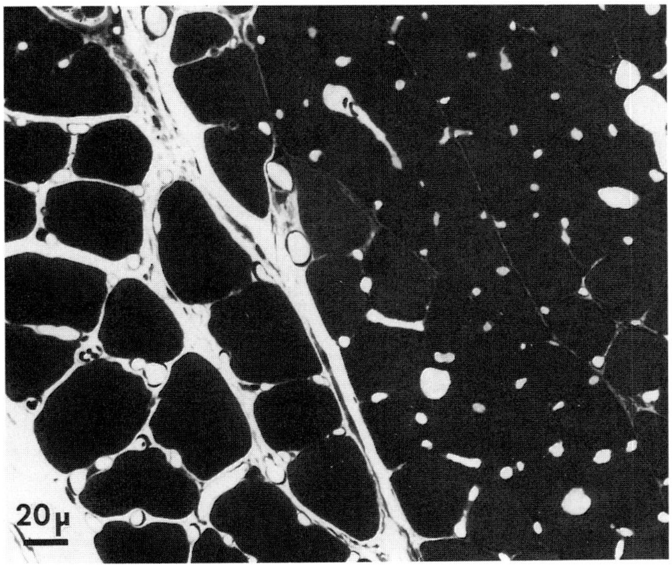

Fig. 8. Light micrograph of portions of two adjacent muscle bundles in transverse section of perfusion-fixed rat soleus muscle. Note the large difference in interfiber spaces within the section, i.e. in portions of tissue subjected to strictly identical preparative steps during fixation, dehydration and tissue embedding for electron microscopy.

Tissue Preparation and Alterations in Capillary Structure

Tissue preparation is obviously critical to morphological studies, and particularly so in studies of ultrastructural damage induced by ischemia or other vascular impairments. Hypoxic cells are known to respond differently to tissue fixatives than normal cells, and they usually require higher fixative osmolarity than normal tissues for adequate ultrastructural preservation. In other words, using the same fixative osmolarity for control and experimental tissues is not necessarily a safeguard against the production of artifacts. For example, Bowers et al. [12] showed that mitochondrial swelling and disruptions found in muscle biopsies after a run to exhaustion were no longer seen, i.e. there was no evidence of mitochondrial damage, when the tissue was fixed with a fixative of higher osmolarity than that used for controls. In such a case, the original finding of mitochondrial abnormality was not totally an artifact, in that changes in the muscle cells and mitochondrial membrane properties occurred after the run to exhaustion, which made the tissue respond differently to the fixative than normal tissue. However, the actual structural disruption of mitochondrial membranes was an artifact. In ultrastructural studies of tissue swelling and disruption, it is important to run fixation tests using solutions with different osmolarities, to dissociate structural changes consequent to physiological changes in the osmotic properties of the tissue, from the actual structural disruption of cells or organelles in the vasculature and surrounding tissue.

Acknowledgments

This work was done in collaboration with Drs. Claire Budreau, Jack G. Copeland, Paul McDonagh, Earl Noble and David C. Poole. Supported by NIH Program Project grant HL-17731, the Heart and Stroke Foundation of Ontario, the Medical Research Council of Canada and the American Heart Association, Arizona Affiliate.

References

1 Armiger LC, Gavin JB: Changes in the microvasculature of ischemic and infarcted myocardium. Lab Invest 1975;33:51–56.

2 Strock PE, Majno G: Microvascular changes in acutely ischemic rat muscle. Surg Gynecol Obstet 1969;129:1213–1224.

3 Gidlöf A, Lewis DH, Hammersen F: The effect of prolonged total ischemia on the ultrastructure of human skeletal muscle capillaries: A morphometric analysis. Int J Microcirc Clin Exp 1987;7:67–86.

4 Tyml K, Mathieu-Costello O, Budreau CH: Microvascular response to ischemia, and tissue structure, in normal and atrophied skeletal muscle. Microvasc Res 1990;39:223–239.

5 Tyml K, Mathieu-Costello O, Budreau CH: Distribution of red blood cell velocity in capillary network, and endothelial ultrastructure, in aged rat skeletal muscle. Microvasc Res 1992;44:1–13.

6 Tyml K, Mathieu-Costello O, Noble E: Microvascular response to ischemia, and endothelial ultrastructure, in disused skeletal muscle. Microvasc Res 1995;49:17–32.

7 Manciet LH, Poole DC, McDonagh PF, Copeland JG, Mathieu-Costello O: Microvascular compression during myocardial ischemia: Mechanistic basis for no-reflow phenomenon. Am J Physiol 1994;266:H1541–H1550.

8 Tyml K, Budreau CH: Heterogeneity of microvascular response to ischemia in skeletal muscle. Int J Microcirc Clin Exp 1988;7:205–221.

9 Tyml K, Budreau CH: A new preparation of rat extensor digitorum longus muscle for intravital investigation of the microcirculation. Int J Microcirc Clin Exp 1991;10:335–343.

10 Mathieu-Costello O: Capillary tortuosity and degree of contraction or extension of skeletal muscles. Microvasc Res 1987;33:98–117.

11 Eisenberg BR, Kuda AM, Peter JB: Stereological analysis of mammalian skeletal muscle. I: Soleus muscle of the adult guinea pig. J Cell Biol 1974;60:732–754.

12 Bowers WD, Hubbard RW, Smoake JA, Daum RC, Nilson E: Effects of exercise on the ultrastructure of skeletal muscle. Am J Physiol 1974;227:313–316.

Int J Microcirc 1995;15:238–243

Amy G. Tsai
Barbara Friesenecker
M. Intaglietta

Department of Bioengineering,
University of California, San Diego,
La Jolla, Calif., USA

Capillary Flow Impairment and Functional Capillary Density

Key Words
Capillary diameter
Capillary contractility
Functional capillary density
Endothelium
Pressure

Abstract
Functional capillary density is variable in both normal and diseased tissue. When this parameter is defined as the number of capillaries that possess red blood cell transit, changes in functional capillary density reflect mechanisms that modulate the entrance of red blood cells into the capillaries. These mechanisms have anatomical origin, whereby the capillary diameter changes, and may also be hydrodynamic, when flow conditions prevent red blood cells from entering a capillary branch. An intrinsic feature of both processes is that capillaries undergo lumenal changes. Capillary lumen is determined by a composite of mechanical and cellular factors, where intravascular pressure is one of the principal determinants affecting diameter as a consequence of the elastic properties of the capillary/tissue system. The hydration of the surrounding tissue and the cellular volume regulation of the endothelium are additional factors. There is increasing evidence that capillaries possess contractility and that this phenomenon has spontaneous components. Consequently, functional capillary density is the resultant of both passive and active processes present at the level of individual vessels.

Introduction

Capillary oxygen delivery is dominated by the large surface area of this vascular compartment and low oxygen gradients. Their small intrinsic oxygen-carrying capacity and low intravascular pO_2 renders each capillary unique in supplying a localized tissue volume, unless this is also within the diffusion field of an arteriole. Consequently, there is a portion of the tissue where capillary flow cessation, i.e., the decrease of functional capillary density, is deleterious and possibly a fatal event.

The mechanism behind changes in the number of capillaries with red blood cell flow has not been demonstrated. Physical considerations suggest that this may result from mechanical events comprising (1) capillary lumen narrowing beyond the point where capillary pressure can provide the energy needed for red blood cell deformation; (2) capillary luminal obstruction by leukocytes, microthrombi, and rigid red blood cells, and (3) hydrodynamic effects at capillary bifurcations which direct red blood cells to the stream with the greater flow and flow velocity. Capillary diameter variability underlies these scenarios, although it is generally assumed that the capillary lumen is mostly invariable and independent of transmural pressure. This perception stems from the conclusion that capillaries are rigid, having the elastic proper-

A.G. Tsai, PhD
Department of Bioengineering
University of California, San Diego
La Jolla, CA 92093-0412 (USA)

ties of the medium in which they are imbedded [1]. It is similarly assumed that they are not contractile.

A corollary to present perceptions of capillary mechanics is that if perfusion pressure decreases, the flow rate decreases throughout the microvascular network, and unless shear rate falls below the yield value for blood (if this obtains in capillary flow), capillary flow should not stop, i.e., there is no change in functional capillary density associated with lowered perfusion pressure.

Studies in the skeletal microcirculation [2] showed that functional capillary density changes reversibly when perfusion pressure varies. Pressure flow studies in isolated organs show that flow hindrance increases as perfusion pressure decreases, a behavior mostly attributed to the shear dependance of blood viscosity and diameter changes in the distensible segments of the vasculature. Decreased functional capillary density has been observed in low-flow conditions associated with ischemia-reperfusion injury [3]. In each case, mechanisms responsible for capillary flow cessation have not been addressed. In this article, we review the mechanical basis associated with capillary red blood cell flow and provide information in support of the concept of active capillary diameter regulation.

Capillary Distensibility and Decompression

Capillary distensibility was studied experimentally by Baez et al. [4] who increased pressure in the rat mesoappendix preparation to 200 mm Hg without detecting diameter changes, thus concluding that these vessels are rigid in the pressure range present in the circulation. Characterization of the capillary mechanical environment by experimental and mathematical modelling in the mesentery showed that they behave like 1 μm wall thickness elastic tubes with 6.8×10^6 dyn/cm^2 wall material modulus, leading to the conclusion that capillary elastic properties are a consequence of the medium in which they are embedded [1].

Independent information on capillary elastic properties was obtained by analyzing the motion of red blood cells in occluded capillaries [5, 6] due to pulsatile pressure [7]. These studies show that after stopping capillary flow by compressing a portion of its length with a microtool, the cells in the portion open to the arterial inflow have oscillatory motion synchronous with the action of the heart. Thus oscillatory behavior of red blood cells in occluded microvessels is due to either the vessel elasticity or to alternating fluid absorption and filtration [7]. The latter requires either large pressure excursions or high permeability, and was excluded in favor of the hypothesis that periodic cell motion was due to vessel distensibility [5].

Most studies analyze the consequence of increasing capillary pressure, rather than the opposite, which occurs if arterial supply is occluded. Capillary pressure in normal conditions is close to the blood colloid osmotic pressure [8], on the order of 30–20 mm Hg: therefore, equilibration to venular/venous pressure reduces by about 10 mm Hg (1.33×10^4 dyn/cm^2). Such a pressure drop causes a diameter reduction given by:

$$\Delta D = \frac{D^2}{2wY} \Delta P, \qquad (1)$$

where D is the inner diameter, w is the capillary wall thickness, ΔP is the pressure change and Y is the modulus of elasticity. Table 1 summarizes lumenal change for a capillary of 8 μm diameter, 1 μm wall thickness, and the different estimates of the Young's modulus for a pressure decrease of 10 mm Hg according to current data. It shows that there are data in support of the concept that modest pressure changes can produce observable diameter variations.

Capillary Dimensions

Considerations of capillary diameter response to changes in internal pressure show discrepancies between results obtained from different methods of study. In terms of capillary decompression, it appears that if we assume that capillaries are highly distensible, the expected pressure changes cannot account for capillary closure provided that the capillary diameter is uniform through its entirety.

Data on individual capillary diameter heterogeneity are scarce and limited to small segments. Analysis of intercapillary diameter nonhomogeneity [13] shows that in skeletal and cardiac muscle, capillary diameter ranges from 2.0 to 10.0 μm, 10% of all capillaries having a diameter less than 3 μm, 2.5% being 2.5 μm or less, and 1.1%, 2.3 μm or less. In this study, diameters were measured at a single location, determinations being made in transversal planes perpendicular to the plane containing the vessels. This approach does not show individual capillary diameter heterogeneity, however, it permits the hypothesis that capillaries may present a diameter heterogeneity similar to intercapillary heterogeneity. In other words, the distribution of capillary diameter between capillaries may be

Table 1. Capillary elastic properties and diameter change for a 10 mm Hg pressure decrease

Method	Reference	Young's modulus dyn/cm²	ΔD, μm (equation 1)
Elastic properties of mesentery (rabbit)	Fung et al. [1]	6.8×10^6	0.06
Phase shift of pulsatile pressure in the microcirculation (rabbit omentum)	Intaglietta et al. [7]	4.5×10^5	0.94
Pulsatile diameter vs. pressure (rabbit omentum capillaries)	Intaglietta et al. [9]	6×10^5	0.71
Red blood cell motion in occluded capillaries (cat mesentery)	Clough et al. [5]		0.2[a]
Red blood cell motion in occluded capillaries (cat mesentery)	Smaje et al. [10]	3.7×10^6	0.12
Motion of oil droplet (frog mesentery)	Swayne et al. [11]	3.4×10^6	0.11
Capillary compliance (frog mesentery)	Smaje et al. [12]		0.6[b]

Nominal diameter = 8 μm, wall thickness of 1 μm.

[a] Calculated.

[b] Estimated from a reported radius change of 1.7% for 2.2 mm Hg pressure change.

similar to the variation in diameter along the capillary length. This is in part supported by the observation that the endothelial cell nucleus often intrudes into the capillary lumen significantly narrowing diameter, an occurrence probably common to each endothelial cell.

If capillaries present significant diameter heterogeneity, it is likely that minimal lumenal narrowing may result in locations that mechanically hinder or prevent red blood cell passage. In narrow capillaries, vessel dimensions and blood viscosity are related [14] and for a capillary diameter below 5 μm, the viscosity increases sharply. This phenomenon is related to the energy required to deform red blood cells past a constriction. The needed energy is provided by the arteriolar/venular pressure gradient and when this is not sufficient, cells do not pass the obstruction, behaving as rigid objects causing viscosity to become infinite. For human blood, the limit to the deformation that cells may undergo corresponds to that necessary to pass through a 2.8 μm diameter tube [10, 15, 16].

Given the hypothesized distribution of capillary nonhomogeneity, some portion of every capillary may be at or near the critical diameter and lower capillary pressures may decrease the lumen causing capillary flow cessation solely due to elastic recoil. Thus, the possibility exists that small diameter reductions have an on-off like control effect on capillary flow.

Endothelial Component of Capillary Lumenal Changes

Capillary diameter is also a function of effects in the cellular lining and endothelial volume. Changes in endothelial configuration and particularly volume are present in ischemia and hemorrhagic shock [3, 17], which cause the influx of sodium and water. Endothelial volume changes can only be accomodated by intrusion into the lumenal compartment and therefore have a profound effect on functional capillary density.

Endothelium has an actin/myosin based contractile system [18] that responds to mediators that also activate smooth muscle cell constriction [19]. Extreme endothelial cell contraction separates cells, increasing capillary permeability; however, this phenomenon has not been related to a decreased capillary lumen.

The existence of an active contractile machinery within the endothelium led Boswell et al. [20] to propose that 'tone', a property assigned to muscular tissue, is present in unitary components of the tissue, at the level of each cell. These cells may exhibit tone of varying degrees in normal conditions. Microvascular studies of arteriolar tone show that in the absence of anesthesia [21], these vessels exhibit a continuous and spontaneous diameter variation, i.e., a continuous modulation of tone. Therefore, if cells such as endothelium, smooth muscle and fibroblasts have tone, we would expect a similar phenomenon to be evident.

As previously discussed, capillary dimensions are such that the optical microscope is severely limited in detecting small variations in diameter. This problem can be circumvented in special capillaries whose diameter is so narrow that red blood cells are either trapped in the lumen, or must deform and assume a cylindrical configuration. Mazzoni et al. [22] measured the lumen by recording the cylindrical axis of the cells as they traversed or became lodged in narrow capillaries. We utilized this technique in the hamster skin fold preparation in normally occurring narrow capillaries and measured the axial length of passing red blood cells. A typical result is shown in figure 1, illustrating lumenal variability as a function of time at a fixed location. These data have two possible interpretations: either there is significant variability in red blood cell volume, or capillary lumen is continuously modulated.

Considering that the apparent variability of length of passing red blood cells is of the order of 20% over a period of several minutes, geometrical considerations indicate that this would correspond to a volume variability of 45% if we assume that there is no change in diameter. This is a rather large variability which favors the interpretation of lumenal modulation.

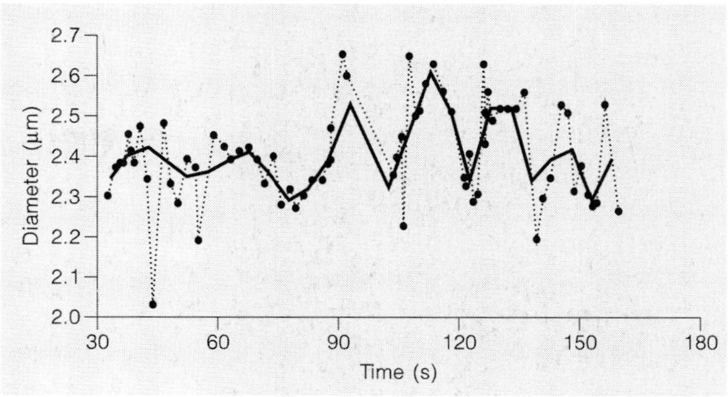

Fig. 1. Variability of diameter in a narrow capillary in the awake hamster skin fold window preparation. Diameter is calculated by assuming that red blood cells have a constant volume. As they traverse narrow capillaries they deform assuming the shape of a cylinder. Measuring the cylinder length allows a determination of capillary diameter. (Broken line = actual data; solid line = moving average). The continuous variability of capillary diameter may be interpreted as evidence that capillaries possess contractile properties and spontaneous activity.

The importance of cellular events that regulate volume and shape of the endothelium is apparent when analyzing hemorrhagic shock, ischemia and reperfusion injury, which lower functional capillary density. Electron microscopy studies and direct in vivo observations of single capillaries during control and reduced or no-flow conditions show that the capillary lumen is reduced while the interstitium is unaltered. These situations are associated with malfunctions in cell volume regulation which present different patterns. In ischemia, the process is sporadic with swollen cells interdispersed with normal cells [17]. In shock, there is a more uniform thickening of the endothelium [3], this latter response being present when endothelial cell cultures are subjected to osmotic transients [23].

Role of the Tissue Compartment

Elasticity of collagen fibrils and glycosaminoglycans provide a tissue structure which opposes deformation of the interstitium by either compression or expansion of the vascular compartment. If capillaries should dilate when capillary pressure increases, the tissue matrix must compress and fluid must be shifted into a tissue reservoir since the compressibility of either is minimal. The only volume reservoir within the tissue that can undergo these types of volumetric changes is the lymphatic compartment, unless there is an overall change of tissue volume. Neither of these effects can be excluded; however, it is unlikely that they play a major role in the absence of conditions that promote massive tissue edema.

In decompression, the vascular compartment is a readily available volume reservoir both as a deposit of extra fluid and as a source of fluid for the changes of tissue volume. In healthy tissue, the change of interstitial volume is due to fluid exchange by the Starling mechanism. When endothelium is intact, blood and tissue compartments are in mechanical balance prior to decompression. When intravascular pressure decreases, fluid exchange is driven by two opposing phenomena: lowering of intravascular pressure that decreases filtration, and lowering of tissue fluid pressure due to tissue decompression which promotes absorption. In this situation, capillaries whose hydrostatic pressure is significantly higher than colloid osmotic pressure, and therefore filter fluid, can decrease their diameter since the necessary fluid may still be forthcoming via filtration from the intravascular space.

There is little information on volume changes of cells that constitute tissue; however, the tissue is regulated to a condition of minimum volume. This is because the net balance of the Starling forces favors absorption of fluid from the tissue space into the blood compartment. The lymphatic system, furthermore, extracts fluids in excess of those managed by the Starling mechanism. Fluid balance is a self-correcting process when absorption favors filtration, since increased negativity of tissue pressure causes the cessation of exchange. When filtration is favored, there is no self-correction because tissue has the capacity to store fluid without increasing tissue pressure, tissue having high compliance in edema. Although tissue edema per se may not influence capillary lumen, many organs are enclosed (muscle by tight fascial sheaths, the brain by the skull) and in the presence of edema this configuration may compress low pressure microvessels, reducing their lumen.

Capillary Hemodynamics and Functional Capillary Density

Functional capillary density is defined in terms of the number of capillaries that present red blood cell flow. Following this definition, it is measured by visually identifying capillaries where red blood transits over periods encompassing naturally occurring flow cessation due to vasomotion. An alternative method is to use plasma markers to delineate the capillaries under the assumption that marker-filled capillaries permit flow. This later method, however, is open to criticism because it may not differentiate between plasma flow and blood flow, which are quite different in terms of oxygen-carrying capacity, since whole blood carries oxygen in a ratio of 71:1 relative to plasma. Consequently, a capillary does not necessarily need to be occluded to be nonfunctional, a condition that may result from conditions that prevent red blood cells from entering a capillary.

It is well established that bifurcating tubes with flow divide the incoming stream into daughter conduits in an inverse proportion to their hydraulic resistance. This process also determines a partition of the flow of the parent vessels according to the streamline that divides the flows, which is positioned closer to the wall on the side of the conduit with slower flow. When particulate matter is present, particles concentrate in the faster moving stream of the lower resistance conduits. In extreme conditions, a very high resistance capillary side branch may only obtain the cell void fluid in the plasma layer, thus producing a nonfunctional capillary.

Hydrodynamic effects of this type yield relatively simple capillary network models where a small variation in diameter due to lowered intravascular pressure produces a significant change of functional capillary density. For instance, a bifurcation with branches of identical hydraulic resistance at normal perfusion pressure but with different diameter and length in each branch, shows a significant increase in hydraulic resistance in the branch with the smaller diameter if decompression affects the whole structure uniformly.

Conclusions

Functional capillary density is related to capillary hemodynamics. Experimental studies to date have not shown the specific mechanism behind this process in vivo. Mechanical considerations indicate that in the absence of cellular events such as leukocyte plugging [24] and thrombosis, the lack of red blood cells in capillaries must arise from filtering effects either due to a decrease in the lumenal diameter below the threshold that allows red blood cell deformation, or hydrodynamic effects in the network. The existence of a spontaneous variability of capillary lumen indicates the potential existence of individual capillary flow regulation through a mechanism intrinsic to endothelial contractility. Pathophysiological conditions may impair endothelial function interfering with local capillary flow regulation, causing endothelial swelling, increased endothelial tone, and increased capillary permeability promoting pericapillary edema. It should be noted that the whole capillary need not necessarily be involved, since only one or a few cells along each capillary intruding into the lumen to the extent that red blood cells cannot pass cause the whole capillary to cease functioning. Capillary perfusion pressure would appear to be the primary factor in determining the extent of functional capillary density. Lowered perfusion pressure coupled to endothelial dysfunction gives rise to the potential for pathological capillary flow hindrance as three mechanisms converge to promote this phenomenon, namely tissue edema, endothelial edema and elastic recoil.

Acknowledgment

The authors thank Ms. Stephanie Oba for data analysis of capillary diameter in the hamster skinfold. This work was supported by a USPHS HLBI grant 48018.

References

1 Fung YC, Zweifach BW, Intaglietta M: Elastic environment of the capillary bed. Circ Res 1966;19:441–461.
2 Lindbom L, Arfors KE: Mechanism and site of control for variation in the number of perfused capillaries in skeletal muscle. Int J Microcirc Clin Exp 1985;4:121–127.
3 Menger MD, Sack FU, Barker JH, Feifel G, Messmer K: Quantitative analysis of microcirculatory disorders after prolonged ischemia in skeletal muscle: Therapeutic effects of prophylactic isovolemic hemodilution. Res Exp Med (Berl) 1988;188:151–166.
4 Baez S, Lamport H, Baez A: Pressure effects in microscopic blood vessels; in Copley AL, Stainsby (eds): Flow Properties of Blood and Other Biological Systems. Oxford, Pergamon, 1960, pp 122–136.
5 Clough G, Fraser PA, Smaje LH: Compliance measurement in single capillaries of the cat mesentery. J Physiol 1974;240(8):1–2.
6 Intaglietta M: Measurement of fluid exchange between single capillaries and tissue in vivo; in Kaley G, Altura B (eds): Microcirculation. Baltimore, University Park Press, 1980, vol 3, pp 393–406.
7 Intaglietta M, Richardson DR, Tompkins WR: Blood pressure, flow, and elastic properties of microvessels of cat omentum. Am J Physiol 1971;221:922–928.
8 Intaglietta M, Zweifach BW: Microcirculatory basis of fluid exchange. Adv Biol Med Phys 1973;15:111–159.
9 Intaglietta M, Tompkins WR: On-line measurement of microvascular dimensions by television microscopy and elastic properties. J Appl Physiol 1972;32:546–551.
10 Smaje LH, Fraser PA, Clough G: The distensibility of single capillaries and venules in the cat mesentery. Microvasc Res 1980;20:358–370.
11 Swayne GTC, Smaje LH, Bergel DH: Distensibility of single capillaries and venules in the rat and frog mesentery. Int J Microcirc Clin Exp 1989;8:25–42.
12 Smaje LH, Swayne GTC: The effects of compliance on measurement of hydraulic conductivity in microvessels. Biorheology 1984;21: 171–179.
13 Potter RF, Groom AC: Capillary diameter and geometry in cardiac and skeletal muscle studied by means of corrosion casts. Microvasc Res 1983;25:68–84.
14 Secomb TW, Fleishman GJ, Papenfuss HD, Intaglietta M, Gross JF: Effects of reduced perfusion and hematocrit on flow distribution in capillary networks. Prog Appl Microcirc 1987; 12:205–211.
15 Henquell L, LaCelle PL, Honig CR: Capillary diameter in rat heart in situ: Relation to erythrocyte deformability, O_2 transport and transmural O_2 gradients. Microvasc Res 1976;12: 259–274.
16 Jay AWL: Viscoelastic properties of human red blood cell membrane. I. Deformation, volume loss, and rupture of red cells in micropipettes. Biophys J 1973;13:1166–1182.
17 Gidlöf A, Lewis DH, Hammersen F: The effect of total ischemia on the ultrastructure of human skeletal muscle capillaries: A morphometric analysis. Int J Microcirc Clin Exp 1987;7: 67–86.
18 Gotlieb AI, Wong MKK: Current concepts on the role of endothelial cytoskeleton in endothelial integrity, repair and dysfunction; in Ryan US (ed): Endothelial Cells. Boca Raton, CRC, 1988, pp 81–101.
19 Boswell CA, Majno G, Joris I, Ostrom KA: Acute endothelial cell contraction in vitro: A comparison with vascular smooth muscle cells and fibroblasts. Microvasc Res 1992;43:178–191.
20 Boswell CA, Joris I, Majno G: The concept of cellular tone: Reflections on the endothelium, fibroblasts and smooth muscle cells. Perspect Biol Med 1992;36:79–86.
21 Colantuoni A, Bertuglia S, Intaglietta M: Effects of anesthesia on the spontaneous activity of the microvasculature. Int J Microcirc Clin Exp 1984;3:13–28.
22 Mazzoni MC, Borgström P, Intaglietta M, Arfors KE: Lumenal narrowing and endothelial cell swelling in skeletal muscle capillaries during hemorrhagic shock. Circ Shock 1989;29: 27–39.
23 Mazzoni MC, Lundgren E, Arfors KE, Intaglietta M: Volume changes of an endothelial cell monolayer on exposure to anisotonic media. J Cell Physiol 1989;140:272–280.
24 Engler RL, Schmid-Schönbein GW, Pavelec RS: Leukocyte capillary plugging in myocardial ischemia and reperfusion in dog. Am J Pathol 1983;111:98–111.

Int J Microcirc 1995;15:244–249

D. Nolte
H. Zeintl
M. Steinbauer
S. Pickelmann
K. Messmer

Institute for Surgical Research, Ludwig Maximilian University, Munich, Germany

Functional Capillary Density: An Indicator of Tissue Perfusion?

Key Words
Hamster
Microcirculation
Heterogeneity
Capillary perfusion
Computer-assisted analysis

Abstract
Functional capillary density (FCD) is one of the parameters obtained by intravital microscopy using epi-illumination of the tissue surface or trans-illumination of thin tissue layers. FCD, defined as the length of red cell-perfused capillaries per observation area (cm^{-1}), has been used as an indicator of the quality of tissue perfusion in various animal models. Quantitative analysis of FCD in randomly selected regions of the tissue is performed by means of a computer-assisted video analysis system which allows calculation of the length of RBC-perfused capillaries. Basically, two different mathematical approaches can be employed: the first approach is based on the addition of the distances between two neighboring points (pixels) on the video screen (Pythagorean principle). The second approach uses the superimposition of a grid system that allows estimation of the capillary length by counting the number of intersections between the capillaries and the grid lines (stereological approach). The immanent error has been calculated in our laboratory to be ± 1% with the Pythagorean and ± 5% with the stereological method. Beside these systematic errors of computerized measurement, the individual (user-dependent) errors occurring during recognition and redrawing of the capillaries on the video image with use of a digitizing tablet are in the range of ± 10% (intraindividual) and ± 70% (interindividual) for the recognition and ± 3% (interindividual) for the redrawing procedure. Our studies indicate that the errors resulting from the use of a computer-assisted calculation (Pythagorean or stereological approach) or the user-assisted redrawing of the capillaries are negligible when compared to the errors made during recognition of the capillaries on the video screen. The methods are applied for assessment of FCD in two different microcirculation models of skin muscle and pancreas yielding highly reproducible, user-independent results under physiologic conditions and the pathophysiologic conditions of ischemia-reperfusion.

Dirk Nolte, MD
Institute for Surgical Research
Klinikum Grosshadern, Marchioninistrasse 15
University of Munich
D-80377 Munich (Germany)

0167–6865/95/0155–0244
$10.00/0

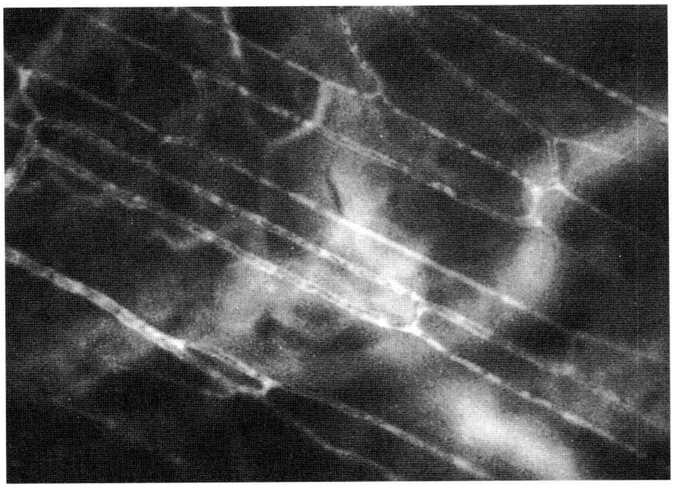

a

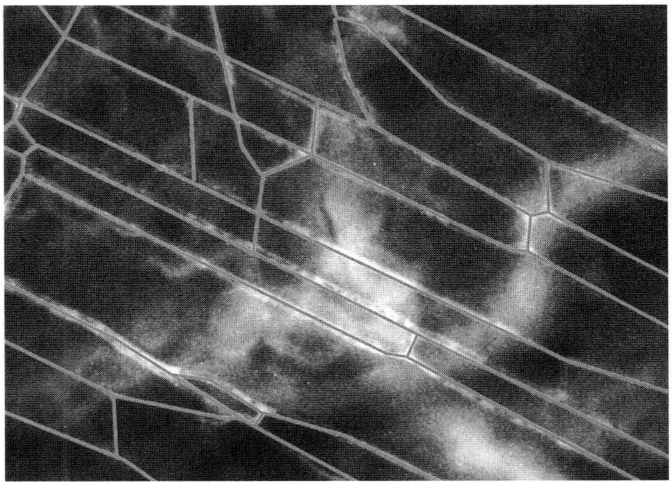

b

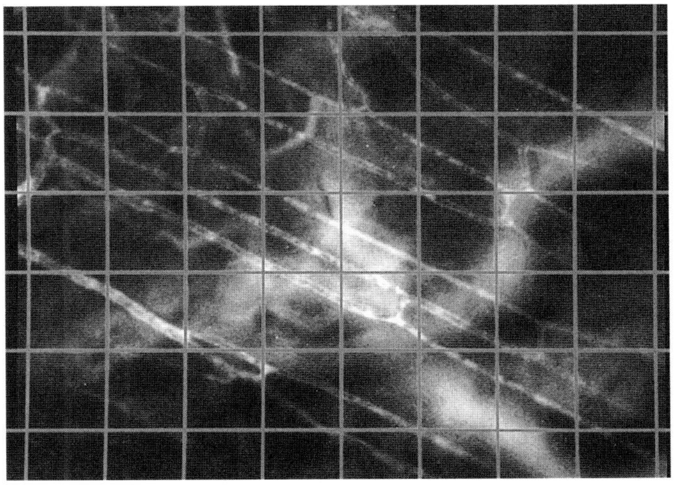

c

Fig. 1. Fluorescence microscopy images of the capillary bed in the striated skin muscle contained within the dorsal skinfold chamber of the Syrian golden hamster. **a** Striated muscle capillaries arranged isotropically with their typical intercapillary connections. For contrast enhancement, plasma (white) is stained with FITC dextran (M_r 150 kD). RBCs are recognizable as plasma gaps (black). × 298. **b** RBC-perfused capillaries are traced with a stylo on the digitizing tablet of the computer-assisted working station. Total capillary length per area is obtained by adding up the straight line elements of all traced lines (Pythagorean principle). **c** Superimposition of a grid system (square type, 75 × 75 μm^2). The number of intersections between perfused capillaries and grid lines serves for estimation of capillary length (stereological principle).

Introduction

Capillary perfusion is a prerequisite for the transport of oxygen, nutrients and metabolites to and from the tissue cells. Therefore, reliable quantification of capillary perfusion represents an important goal of experimental and clinical research. The nutritive perfusion of a tissue depends on the number and anatomical distribution of capillaries and on the blood flow within these conduits. As a quantitative parameter, functional capillary density (FCD) has been proposed as a measure of capillary perfusion under various pathophysiological circumstances such as ischemia-reperfusion [1–10], pancreatitis [11–13] and shock [14].

Since capillaries cannot simply be regarded as tubes running straight and unbranched as assumed in the capillary model of Krogh [15, 16], various investigators aimed at the calculation of this parameter by means of stereological methods in order to account for the spatial geometry of the capillary network [17, 18]. This approach is based on the evaluation of tissue sections which have to be cut longitudinally and transsectionally to the direction of the capillaries. Using intravital fluorescence microscopy and the dorsal skinfold model in hamsters and mice [5, 19, 20], two-dimensional images of capillary networks are provided which reflect the projection of tissue sections of 250 µm thickness and 450 µm length. Figure 1 shows such a videotaped image obtained from the striated skin muscle in the hamster skinfold chamber (fig. 1a). Although the capillary density obtained from this image does not take into account the spatial arrangement of the depicted capillaries as achieved by the stereological method, this approach gives the number of capillaries more accurately than to be obtained from a transsectional cut.

In the following, the term 'functional capillary density' is used as capillary length per observation area and expressed as cm^{-1}; the term 'functional' capillary density (FCD) is restricted to the analysis of the RBC-perfused capillaries.

A method for manual calculation of capillary density is based on the stereological concept that has been described by Schmid-Schoenbein et al. [21]. It requires the superimposition of a grid system onto the video image (fig. 1c). However, this method requires the montage of many single video images to an entire capillary network and is therefore very time-consuming, highly expensive (costs for photomaterial) and relatively imprecise. From the number of intersections (N) per total length of the grid lines (L_G) an estimation for capillary density (CD) can be calculated according to the formula: $CD = (\Pi/2) \cdot (N/L_G)$.

In order to facilitate the analysis of CD, the computer-assisted microcirculation analysis system, CAMAS, has been developed in our laboratory for rapid recognition and evaluation of intravital microscopic images [22]. The total length of all capillaries is calculated by the computer through addition of the distances assessed between two neighboring points on the video screen (pixels). The length of such a single partial line (dL) is calculated by the Pythagorean formula (see below). The problem arising from this approach of calculation concerns the precision of the measurement since, instead of directly measuring a continuous straight line, the total length of the line is calculated by adding the single partial lines yielding a step-shaped curve which is due to the pixel composition of the video image. However, the error immanent in this approach can be reduced by adequate modifying measures.

Besides these problems inherent to the computer-assisted calculation of the capillary length, individual (user-dependent) errors are made in recognizing microvascular structures on the video screen as capillaries per se and, moreover, as functional, i.e. RBC-perfused, capillaries. Furthermore, the impact of errors made during the redrawing of the recognized capillaries on the digitizing tablet have to be taken into account when absolute values for FCD are to be gained.

Herein, we report on some basic considerations that have to be taken into account for the evaluation of FCD by computer-assisted video analysis systems with focus on both system-immanent and individual (user-dependent) errors. The biological meaning of FCD as an indicator of microvascular tissue perfusion is analyzed under both physiological and pathophysiological conditions in two different microcirculation models.

Material and Methods

Animal Models

Intravital fluorescence microscopy was performed in the microcirculation of (1) the striated skin muscle of conscious Syrian golden hamsters [4, 19] and mice [5, 20, 23], and (2) the pancreas of male Sprague-Dawley rats [11]. Both models permit the intravital microscopic investigation of microhemodynamic parameters, including vessel diameter and red cell velocity, as well as quantitative assessment of leukocyte-endothelial cell interactions, macromolecular leakage, and FCD [4, 11].

Intravital Fluorescence Microscopy

A 25-fold water immersion lens (total magnification 560-fold; E. Leitz, Inc., Wetzlar, Germany) was used to select the regions of interest for the assessment of FCD. For fluorescent capillaroscopy, the plasma was stained with fluorescein isothiocyanate-labelled dextran (FITC dextran, 15 mg × kg^{-1} body weight, M_r 150,000, Pharmacia, Uppsala, Sweden). FCD, which is defined as the length of RBC-perfused capillaries per observation area and expressed in cm^{-1}, was assessed in the striated skin muscle of the hamster by the Pythagorean quantification using the Computer-Assisted Microcirculation Analysis System (CAMAS) [24] and in the pancreas by a stereological approach according to the method described by Schmid-Schoenbein et al. [21].

Mathematical Approaches for the Calculation of the Length of Perfused Capillaries

The Pythagorean Principle. This method is based on the addition of partial lines (dL) assessed between two neighboring pixels on the video screen and is calculated according to the Pythagorean formula:

$$dL = \sqrt{(dx^2 + dy^2)}.$$

The approach is commonly used in digital image analysis systems for calculation of the length of a line [25]. Instead of measuring the real length of a line on the video screen, the computer calculates the length in the form of a step-shaped line, which is significantly longer than the real line. Therefore, various methods have been developed to reduce this mathematical error, which is due to the finite solution of the video screen. For this purpose, either the corner points are omitted during calculation (measure a), or omission of corner points plus of every third point on the step line (measure b), or omission of the corner points plus three-point smoothening of the x and y coordinates are performed (measure c) [22, 26].

Stereological Principle. This method employs statistical approaches to determine the geometrical structure of an object on the basis of the knowledge of a representative part of the total structure. The stereological method applied for the calculation of CD uses a grid that is superimposed on the video image (fig. 1c). From the number of intersections (N) per total length of the grid lines (L_G) an estimation for CD can be performed according to the stereological formula. The details of the mathematical derivation of this approach both for isotropic and anisotropic structures has been described by Weibel [27, 28].

Table 1. Functional capillary density (FCD) of striated skin muscle in the dorsal skinfold chamber model of hamster and mouse

Species	Condition	FCD, cm^{-1}	Authors
Hamster	awake	179 ± 35	Franke et al. [29]
Hamster	pentobarbital anesthesia	131 ± 30	Franke et al. [29]
Hamster	enflurane anesthesia	210 ± 45	Endrich et al. [30]
Hamster	awake	160 ± 10	Lehr et al. [2]
Hamster	awake	175 ± 15	Nolte et al. [6]
Hamster	awake	180 ± 20	Menger et al. [3]
Hamster	awake	141 ± 25	Sirsjö et al. [9]
Hamster	awake	156 ± 19	Harris et al. [1]
Hamster	awake	148 ± 22	Steinbauer et al. [10]
Hamster	awake	153 ± 21	Pickelmann et al. [8]
Hamster	awake	131 ± 31	Botzlar et al. [14]
SCID mouse	awake	295 ± 33	Leunig et al. [22]
Nude mouse	awake	249 ± 12	Lehr et al. [20]
Balb/c mouse	awake	220 ± 20	Nolte et al. [5]

Values are mean ± SD analyzed under physiologic conditions.

Results and Discussion

Methodological Considerations

The Pythagorean approach for calculation of the length yields maximal errors up to 41.4% if no correction measure (see Methods) for improvement of precision is used. Measure a (omission of corner points) yields a maximal error of 13.4%, measure b (omission of corner points plus omission of every third point on the step line) and measure c (omission of corner points plus three-point smoothening of x and y coordinates) each yield a maximum error of 2.7% when rectangular pixels are used. These errors can be reduced to 35.2% if no measure is applied, 8.2% with measure a, and 1.3% with both measures b and c when quadrangular pixels are used [22].

The immanent errors in calculating the length according to the Pythagorean principle can be diminished to a tolerable degree when measures b and c are implemented. Both measures provide similar results which can furthermore be reduced by the mean standard error of deviation to ± 1%.

In the case of the stereological method the observed errors based on the isotropy formula yield acceptable results in the presence of isotropy (± 5%). In the case of partial or complete anisotropy, a considerable scattering from −22 to +15% has been found for anisotropic structures. However, it could be demonstrated that the scattering of the results with each degree of anisotropy and with all angles of the preferred direction remains below ± 5%. Hence, the stereological formula yields results within an error being < ± 5%, thus providing acceptable precision also for anisotropic structures.

Taken together, the investigations from our laboratory have demonstrated that the error of calculation of the capillary length using computer-assisted digital video analysis is < ± 1% for the Pythagorean approach and < ± 5% for the stereological approach. These errors, along with the error for redrawing the capillaries on the video screen using the digitizing tablet, which is in the range of ± 3% for interindividual and ± 1.5% for intraindividual analysis, are negligible when compared to the error arising from the capillary recognition process. Depending on the investigator, this error amounts to ± 10% for experienced but up to 70% for inexperienced investigators. Our results demonstrate that the combination of a manual (capillary recognition) and a half-automated method (computer-assisted calculation of capillary length) which requires the recognition process by man are not suitable for calculation of CD. Therefore, a fully automated method that integrates both capillary recognition and calculation of length independent of the investigator has been developed in our laboratory [22].

Biological Considerations

Numerous studies from our laboratory have investigated CD as a 'functional' parameter to describe the quality of nutritive perfusion of the tissue under both physiologic and pathophysiologic conditions in various organs (table 1–3). The fact that different investigators came up with comparable values of FCD for different organs

Table 2. Functional capillary density (FCD) in the dorsal skinfold chamber model of hamsters and mice after ischemia reperfusion (mean ± SD)

Species	Type of ischemia	Baseline FCD, cm⁻¹	0.5-hour reperfusion		Authors
			FCD, cm⁻¹	% of baseline	
Hamster	tourniquet	180 ± 20	80 ± 40[1]	44[1]	Menger et al. [3]
Hamster	pressure	160 ± 10	95 ± 25	60	Lehr et al. [2]
Hamster	pressure	175 ± 15	100 ± 10	57	Nolte et al. [6]
Hamster	pressure	186 ± 12	83 ± 44	45	Harris et al. [1]
Hamster	pressure	148 ± 22	63 ± 45	43	Steinbauer et al. [10]
Balb/c mouse	pressure	220 ± 20	120 ± 40[2]	55[2]	Nolte et al. [5]

If not otherwise indicated, a 4-hour ischemia was induced followed by 0.5-hour reperfusion.
[1] 1-Hour reperfusion.
[2] 3-Hour ischemia.

Table 3. Functional capillary density (FCD) of exocrine pancreas in rats (mean ± SD)

Baseline FCD, cm⁻¹	Insult	FCD, cm⁻¹		Authors
		1 h after insult	2 h after insult	
360 ± 30	taurocholate-pancreas	250 ± 30	210 ± 15	Kerner et al. [13]
407 ± 24	2-hour ischemia	210 ± 32	140 ± 74	Hoffmann et al. [11]
408 ± 25	2-hour ischemia	200 ± 13	160 ± 27	Hoffmann et al. [12]

(striated skin muscle, pancreas) indicates that this parameter can be reproducibly assessed with the currently available system [24]. FCD is used as an important quality criterion to include or exclude animal preparations from our experiments. FCD values at baseline that are far below the normal range (table 1–3) are indicative of trauma during surgery or surgical exposure of the preparation (pancreas). As a rule, we find in these cases an enhancement of intravascular leukocyte/endothelium interaction in postcapillary venules. It should be noted that FCD, defined as the length of RBC-perfused capillaries per observation area, cannot be understood as a parameter directly indicative of blood supply to the tissue since the RBC velocity in perfused capillaries, known to crucially affect local tissue oxygen tension [31], may be significantly different in individual capillaries.

A constant finding under the conditions of ischemia-reperfusion of striated skin muscle in the hamster is, independent of the investigator, the significant decrease in FCD in the early reperfusion period by about 50% (table 2). Similar findings were obtained after ischemia-reperfusion of murine striated skin muscle [5]. Slight differences in the extent of capillary perfusion failure have been detected with use of this parameter when a 4-hour tourniquet ischemia is compared to a 4-hour pressure-induced ischemia. The lower values of FCD after pressure-induced ischemia have to be attributed, at least in part, to the additional mechanical compression of the capillaries during ischemia [7]. When quantitative analysis of FCD is performed before and after an ischemia of 2 h duration to the exocrine pancreas of the rat, a similar reduction in FCD of about 50% is observed while the chemical insult of a taurocholate-induced pancreatitis yields a markedly less pronounced reduction in FCD (table 3).

We conclude that FCD is a useful indicator of the quality of capillary perfusion under both physiological and pathophysiological conditions. By using today's Cap-Image® System (Dr. Zeintl, Heidelberg, Germany), FCD can be determined with high precision and reproducibility.

References

1 Harris AG, Leiderer R, Messmer K: Skeletal muscle microvascular and tissue injury after varying durations of ischemia. Am J Physiol 1996, in press.

2 Lehr HA, Guhlmann A, Nolte D, Keppler D, Messmer K: Preservation of postischemic capillary perfusion by selective inhibition of leukotriene biosynthesis. Transplant Proc 1991;23: 833–834.

3 Menger MD, Sack FU, Barker JH, Feifel G, Messmer K: Quantitative analysis of microcirculatory disorders after prolonged ischemia in skeletal muscle. Therapeutic effects of prophylactic isovolemic hemodilution. Res Exp Med (Berl) 1988;188:151–165.

4 Nolte D, Bayer M, Lehr HA, Becker M, Krombach F, Kreimeier U, Messmer K: Attenuation of postischemic microvascular disturbances in striated muscle by hyperosmolar saline dextran. Am J Physiol 1992;263:H1411–H1416.

5 Nolte D, Hecht R, Schmid P, et al: Role of Mac-1 and ICAM-1 in ischemia reperfusion injury in a microcirculation model of BALB/C mice. Am J Physiol 1994;36:H1320–H1328.

6 Nolte D, Lehr HA, Sack FU, Messmer K: Reduction of postischemic reperfusion injury by the vasoactive drug buflomedil. Blood Vessels 1991;28(suppl 1):8–14.

7 Nolte D, Menger MD, Messmer K: Microcirculatory models of ischemia-reperfusion injury in skin and striated muscle. Int J Microcirc Clin Exp 1995;15(suppl 1):9–16.

8 Pickelmann S, Nolte D, Messmer K: Effects of diaspirin crosslinked hemoglobin (DCLHb) on postischemic leukocyte/endothelium interaction in striated muscle of the hamster (abstract). Int J Microcirc Clin Exp 1996, in press.

9 Sirsjö A, Lehr HA, Nolte D, Haapaniemi T, Lewis DH, Nylander G, Messmer K: Hyperbaric oxygen treatment enhances the recovery of blood flow and functional capillary density in postischemic striated muscle. Circ Shock 1993;40:9–13.

10 Steinbauer M, Harris AG, Messmer K: Effects of various molecular weight dextrans on microvascular ischemia-reperfusion injury in striated muscle. Am J Physiol 1995, in press.

11 Hoffmann TF, Leiderer R, Waldner H, Messmer K: Ischemia-reperfusion of the pancreas: A new in vivo model for acute pancreatitis in rats. Res Exp Med (Berl) 1995;195:125–144.

12 Hoffmann TF, Uhl E, Messmer K: Protective effect of the somatostatin analogue octreotide in ischemia/reperfusion-induced acute pancreatitis in rats. Pancreas 1996, in press.

13 Kerner T, Vollmar B, Menger MD, Waldner H, Messmer K: Pancreatic microcirculation in acute pancreatitis in rats: Effects of hypotension, crystalloid volume and hemodilution. J Surg Res 1996, in press.

14 Botzlar A, Nolte D, Messmer K: Resuscitation from severe hemorrhagic shock with ultrapurified bovine hemoglobin (U-PBHb): Effects on the microcirculation of striated muscle (abstract). Int J Microcirc Clin Exp 1996, in press.

15 Krogh A: The supply of oxygen to the tissue and the regulation of the capillary circulation. J Physiol 1919;52:457–474.

16 Krogh A: The number and distribution of capillaries in muscles with calculations of the oxygen pressure head necessary for supplying the tissue. J Physiol 1919;52:409–415.

17 Mathieu O, Cruz-Orive LM, Hoppeler H, Weibel ER: Estimating length density and quantifying anisotropy in skeletal muscle capillaries. J Microsc 1983;131:131–146.

18 James NT: A stereological analysis of capillaries in normal and hypertrophic muscle. J Morphol 1981;168:43–49.

19 Endrich B, Asaishi K, Götz A, Messmer K: Technical report: A new chamber technique for microvascular studies in unanesthetized hamsters. Res Exp Med (Berl) 1980;177:125–134.

20 Lehr HA, Leunig M, Menger MD, Nolte D, Messmer K: Dorsal skinfold chamber technique for intravital microscopy in nude mice. Am J Pathol 1993;143:1055–1062.

21 Schmid-Schoenbein GW, Zweifach BW, Kovalchek S: The application of stereological principles to morphometry of the microcirculation in different tissues. Microvasc Res 1977; 14:303–317.

22 Zeintl H: Computergestützte Kapillarerkennung und Kapillardichtebestimmung in der Intravitalmikroskopie; PhD thesis Unversity of Heidelberg, 1985.

23 Leunig M, Yuan F, Menger MD, Boucher Y, Goetz AE, Messmer K, Jain RK: Angiogenesis, microvascular architecture, microhemodynamics, and interstitial fluid pressure during early growth of human adenocarcinoma LS174T in SCID mice. Cancer Res 1992;52: 6553–6560.

24 Zeintl H, Sack F-U, Intaglietta M, Messmer K: Computer-assisted leukocyte velocity measurement in intravital microscopy. Int J Microcirc Clin Exp 1989;8:293–302.

25 Freeman H, Guerrieri E: CHAP: A transportable line-drawing software package. Proc 6th Int Conf on Pattern Recognition, Munich, Oct. 19–22, 1976, pp 79–82.

26 Paul J, Exner HE: Effectivity of effector systems and perimeter algorithms for automatic image analysis. Proc 3rd Eur Symp for Stereology, Ljubljana, June 22–26, 1981, pp 189–198.

27 Weibel ER: Stereological Methods. Vol 1. London, Academic Press, 1979.

28 Weibel ER: Stereological Methods. Vol 2. London, Academic Press, 1980.

29 Franke N, Endrich B, Laubenthal H, Peter K, Messmer K: The effect of pentobarbital on the microcirculation of skeletal muscles and the subcutis. An animal-experimental study. Anästh Intensivther Notfallmed 1982;17:11–14.

30 Endrich B, Franke N, Peter K, Messmer K: Induced hypotension: Action of sodium nitroprusside and nitroglycerin on the microcirculation. A micropuncture investigation. Anesthesiology 1987;66:605–613.

31 Kerger H, Torres IP, Rivas M, Winslow RM, Intaglietta M: Systemic and subcutaneous microvascular oxygen tension in conscious Syrian golden hamsters. Am J Physiol 1995;37:H802–H810.

Int J Microcirc 1995;15:250–254

T.W. Secomb
R. Hsu

Department of Physiology,
University of Arizona, Tucson, Ariz., USA

Red Blood Cell Mechanics and Functional Capillary Density

Key Words
Microcirculation
Blood flow
Red blood cells
Capillaries
Functional capillary density
Blood rheology

Abstract
The relationship between red blood cell mechanics and functional capillary density is examined. Experimental observations of capillary recruitment in skeletal muscle have shown sequential recruitment and derecruitment of capillaries fed by a single arteriole, implying that flow may cease in individual capillaries at small nonzero driving pressures. Such behavior is not expected in uniform blood-perfused tubes, but could occur when moving red cells encounter geometrical irregularities in capillaries. From known elastic properties of the red cell membrane, a lower bound is computed for the pressure required to sustain red cell motion in irregular capillaries. This may be an underestimate of the pressure required, because it neglects the viscous resistance of the red cell membrane when it undergoes transient deformations. Simulations including membrane viscosity show that viscous effects can substantially increase flow resistance. It is concluded that the mechanical properties of red blood cells can play a significant role in the modulation of functional capillary density.

Introduction

Oxygen supply to skeletal muscle is strongly dependent on the functional capillary density, i.e., on the number of capillaries containing a moving stream of red blood cells, per unit cross-sectional area of muscle. With exercise and other types of stimulation, recruitment of capillaries (increase in functional capillary density) occurs, increasing the oxygen supply to the muscle. The existence of capillary recruitment has long been known, but its mechanisms remain incompletely understood. Krogh [1] presented evidence that active changes of capillary diameters are responsible. This view has not been generally accepted, since spontaneous contractions of capillary endothelial cells have not been observed in mammalian skeletal muscle, although spontaneous contractions of capillaries have been observed in spleens of rats and mice [2]. Instead, the prevalent view is that the number of functional capillaries in mammalian skeletal muscle is dictated mainly by the constriction or dilation of arterioles [3, 4]. Each arteriole modulates the flow in an associated group of capillaries fed by it [5].

According to this view, simultaneous recruitment of all capillaries fed by a given arteriole might be expected, upon dilation of the arteriole. However, this is not necessarily the case. Using the rabbit tenuissimus, Lindbom and Arfors [6] showed sequential starts of flow in capillaries fed by a single arteriole, as the arteriole dilated in response to reduced oxygen levels. Decreasing perfusion pressure led to flow cessation in capillaries in almost exactly the reverse sequence. According to these observations, capillary recruitment can occur in several steps, even among the capillaries fed by a single arteriole. The number of perfused capillaries is a function of the pressure gradient acting over the capillary bed, which depends on the degree of contraction of the arteriole [6]. Flow in each capillary ceases when the driving pressure falls below a minimum level or 'yield stress', which varies from one capillary to another. Delashaw and Duling [7], using the hamster tibialis anterior muscle, observed that flow cessa-

Dr. T.W. Secomb
Department of Physiology
University of Arizona
Tucson, AZ 85724 (USA)

tion in capillaries fed by a single arteriole usually occurred simultaneously during gradual arteriolar constriction. However, sequential flow cessation was observed in about 13% of the capillary networks studied.

The above observations imply that flow may cease in individual capillaries in the presence of a nonzero driving pressure. The object of this paper is to examine possible mechanisms for such flow cessation. Lindbom and Arfors [6] observed no change in capillary diameters during the procedures described above, implying that capillaries remained patent throughout, and that cellular elements of the blood are involved in flow cessation. They deduced that the pressure level at which flow ceases depends on the 'length, diameter, geometry, number of red cells and occasional presence of white cells within the vessel'. White cells are certainly capable of blocking flow in capillaries at positive driving pressures, but they are not present in sufficient numbers to account for the observed sequential flow cessation. Therefore, the focus here is on the mechanics of red cell motion and deformation in capillaries and the role of red cells in determining functional capillary density.

Mechanical Properties of Red Blood Cells

The mechanical properties of mammalian red blood cells have been studied extensively [8, 9]. A thin viscoelastic membrane surrounds the cytoplasm. Its elastic shear modulus (about 0.006 dyn/cm in humans) is several orders of magnitude lower than the modulus of isotropic dilation (about 500 dyn/cm) and so the membrane shears readily but resists area changes. Also, bending resistance is small, about 1.8×10^{-12} dyn·cm [10]. A Kelvin solid model can be used for the viscoelastic behavior of the membrane, with the total stress represented as the sum of viscous and elastic contributions [11].

As a result of its fluid interior and the low resistance of its membrane to shear and bending deformations, a red cell is highly deformable, as long as changes in surface area or volume are not required. This allows it to pass through capillaries with diameters much less than its unstressed diameter (8 μm in humans). However, the incompressibility of the interior and the strong resistance of the membrane to area changes imply a minimum diameter for cylindrical tubes that will permit a red cell to pass through intact. For a typical human red cell, this diameter is about 2.8 μm [12, 13]. If a microvessel constricts to a diameter very close to this, red cells are unable to pass even at high driving pressures, and flow ceases. Such constrictions are observed in terminal arterioles [14]. However, evidence already described implies that flow may cease at small nonzero driving pressures in capillaries with diameters well above the critical value. The conditions under which such flow cessation could occur are considered below.

Motion of Red Blood Cells in Uniform Microvessels

Knowledge of the mechanical properties of red blood cells provides a basis for theoretical models of the motion of red cells in uniform microvessels. Single-file motion, as can occur in capillaries with diameters of about 6 μm or less, is particularly amenable to analysis. Models have been developed for this case, assuming axisymmetric geometry, using lubrication theory to describe the plasma flow around the cells, and including the elastic response of the cell membrane to shear and bending deformations [13, 15–17]. These models lead to predictions of the resistance to flow in uniform cylindrical tubes, as a function of tube diameter, hematocrit and cell velocity. Resistance is expressed in terms of apparent viscosity μ_{app}, the viscosity of a Newtonian fluid that would result in the same flow rate according to Poiseuille's law for the same vessel geometry and driving pressure. In single-file flow, apparent viscosity depends linearly on hematocrit:

$$\mu_{app} = \mu_p (1 + K_T H_T)$$

where μ_p is the plasma viscosity, H_T is the tube hematocrit and K_T, the 'apparent intrinsic viscosity', depends on diameter and cell velocity.

Figure 1 shows the predicted variation of K_T with velocity, for tube diameters of 4 and 6 μm. (The slight irregularity of the predicted values near 0.1 cm/s is a result of a change in the computational method at this value.) For velocities above about 0.1 cm/s, K_T is relatively low. At velocities below 0.1 cm/s, however, K_T increases substantially with decreasing velocity, because the lubricating plasma layer around each cell becomes increasingly narrow. The question arises whether this increasing flow resistance could result in flow cessation at a positive driving pressure. In that case, driving pressure would be almost independent of cell velocity at very low velocities, implying that K_T would vary as $(\text{velocity})^{-1}$. As figure 1 indicates, the actual predicted variation of K_T is weaker, approximately as $(\text{velocity})^{-0.4}$. Therefore, flow cessation at positive driving pressures is *not* predicted by these models.

Effects of Microvessel Nonuniformity

In reality, capillaries have irregular and nonuniform cross sections [18, 19]. To pass through a region of local reduction in the capillary cross section, a red cell must usually undergo a transient deformation. The pressure required to drive the cell at a given velocity is then larger, since the viscous and elastic resistance of the cell to deformation must be overcome, in addition to the viscosity of the plasma surrounding the cell. If the driving pressure is insufficient, flow may cease. Here, we first analyze the consequences of cell membrane elasticity, and then consider the influence of viscous effects.

The elastic energy associated with red cell membrane deformation in capillaries can be estimated from theoretical models of red cell motion in uniform tubes [16]. This deformational energy increases from 0.1×10^{-9} erg to 2.5×10^{-9} erg as tube diameter is decreased from 8 to 4 μm. An order-of-magnitude calculation [16] indicates the conditions under which flow cesssation might be expected. Suppose that a cell flowing along a 5-μm capillary encounters a localized constriction, equivalent to a 1-μm reduction in diameter, and occurring over one cell length (7.5 μm). The increase in elastic energy associated with a reduction in diameter from 5 to 4 μm is 1.3×10^{-9} erg. This implies that a pressure difference of at least 9 dyn/cm^2 across the cell is required to allow it to pass the constriction. Flow ceases if the available pressure is less than this level, which is comparable to the expected pressure drop acting along uniform capillaries at very low flow rates. For instance, consider a uniform tube, with diameter 5 μm and length 100 μm, containing four red cells, corresponding to a tube hematocrit of 0.18. If the cells are moving with velocity 0.01 mm/s, the pressure drop is 40 dyn/cm^2, based on $K_T = 10$, from figure 1.

The effects of flow cessation by this mechanism in a network have been simulated [20]. Flow in a capillary network in the cat sartorius muscle [21] was modeled, taking into account the rheological behavior of blood in uniform capillary tubes and the unequal partition of hematocrit at bifurcations. The capillaries entering and leaving the network were considered to be attached to identical networks on either side, so that the network analyzed formed part of an array of repeating units extending along the muscle. The effects of irregularities in capillary cross section were simulated by calculating the minimum pressure drop required for a red cell to pass a 1-μm constriction. If the pressure drop along a capillary segment, divided by the number of cells, was less than this minimum value, then flow was considered to cease in that segment, which was excluded form the network. This procedure was repeated until every remaining segment had a sufficient pressure drop to ensure red cell motion, for a given rate of blood flow into the network.

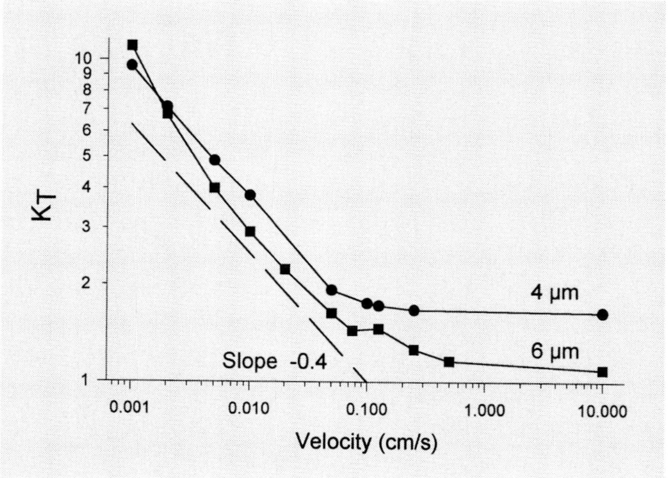

Fig. 1. Predicted variation with cell velocity of apparent intrinsic viscosity K_T in uniform tubes with diameters of 4 and 6 μm. --- = Slope of –0.4.

Simulations were performed for a decreasing sequence of network flows. When the flow velocity in the feeding arteriole fell below about 0.04 cm/s, flow cessation was predicted in an increasing number of segments. Examples are shown in figure 2, and the results are summarized in figure 3. Qualitatively, the behavior observed experimentally [6] is apparent in the simulations. However, the predicted capillary velocities below which flow ceases are of the order of 0.002 cm/s, significantly lower than observed. This suggests that the minimum pressure required to sustain flow through irregular capillaries may be larger than the above estimates.

Several effects which are neglected in the above simulations may contribute to this discrepancy. First, the membrane exhibits viscous resistance to transient shear deformations. Second, the lubricating plasma layer may become thinner when a red cell encounters an obstacle, increasing viscous resistance to flow. Third, low driving pressures may result in a slight decrease in capillary diameter, as a result of capillary compliance.

To investigate the effects of membrane viscosity and thinning of the lubricating plasma layer, we developed a preliminary model for transient motions of red cells in capillaries with variable cross sections. As before, axisymmetric cell shapes are assumed, and lubrication theory is used. In this preliminary model, the elastic resistance of

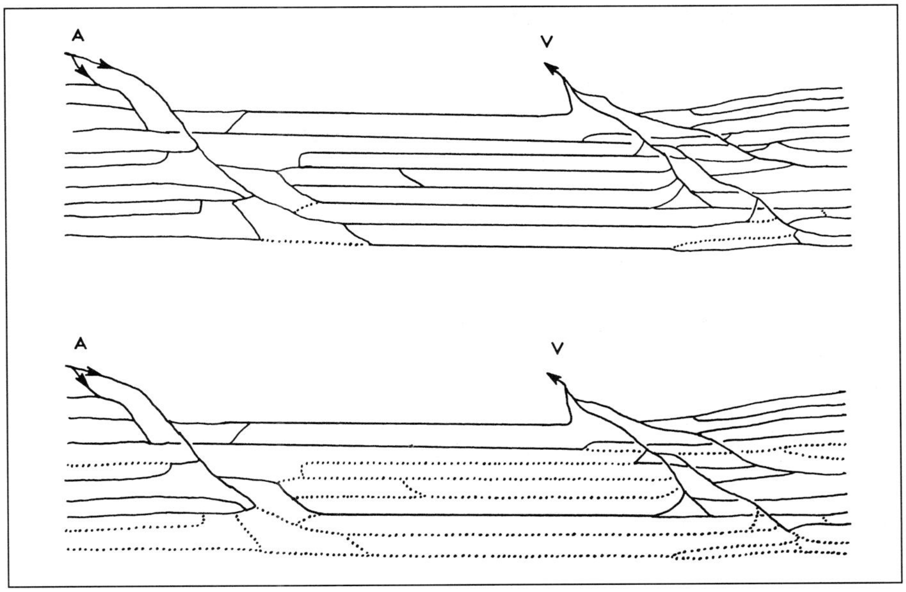

Fig. 2. Maps of a capillary network in cat sartorius, showing predicted flowing segments (—) and nonflowing segments (······) [20]. Arteriolar inflow velocity = 0.02 cm/s (upper) and 0.01 cm/s (lower).

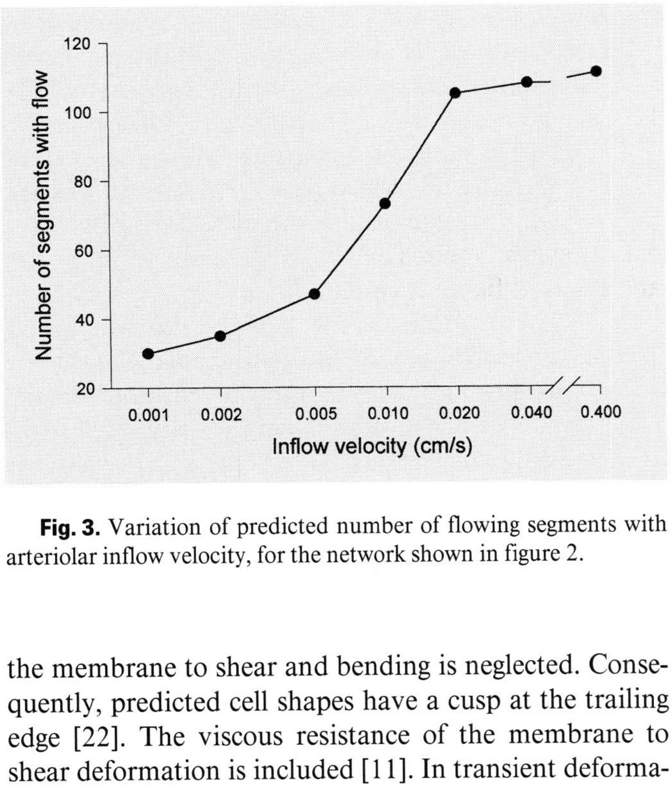

Fig. 3. Variation of predicted number of flowing segments with arteriolar inflow velocity, for the network shown in figure 2.

the membrane to shear and bending is neglected. Consequently, predicted cell shapes have a cusp at the trailing edge [22]. The viscous resistance of the membrane to shear deformation is included [11]. In transient deformations, gap widths vary with time, leading to a time-dependent lubrication equation. This equation, and the equations of equilibrium of normal and tangential forces on the membrane, are solved numerically by a finite-difference method [23].

Figure 4 shows an example in which a red cell in a 7-μm tube encounters a local reduction in tube diameter to

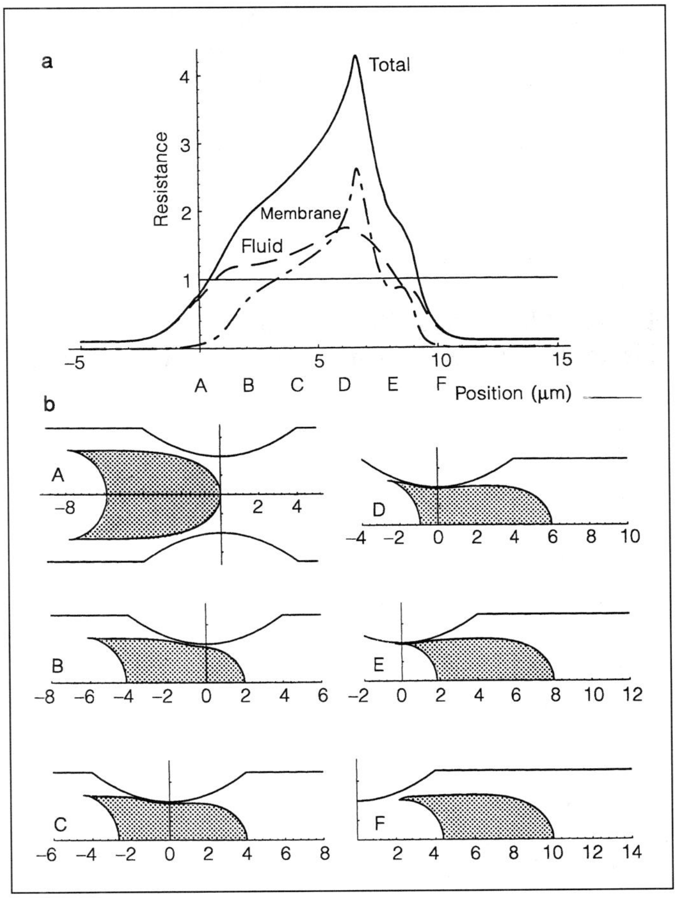

Fig. 4. Simulations of transient red cell deformation in a capillary with a localized constriction. **a** Flow resistance as a function of position, relative to flow resistance in a uniform 4-μm tube (horizontal line), showing contributions of fluid and membrane dissipation to the total. **b** Cell shapes at several positions, denoted A–F. Horizontal scale in μm.

4 μm, representing, for instance, a bulging endothelial nucleus. The flow resistance is proportional to the rate of viscous energy dissipation, which may be expressed as the sum of contributions from the membrane and from the lubrication layer. As the cell begins to squeeze through the constriction, the membrane is deformed, and the width of the lubrication layer is reduced. Total resistance to flow increases to more than fourfold the resistance that the cell would experience in a uniform 4-μm tube. Similar behavior is seen when a red cell enters a narrow capillary from a larger vessel, as at a capillary bifurcation [23]. Thus, irregularities in capillary geometry may contribute substantially to flow resistance, as proposed previously [24]. In this model, which neglects cell elasticity, flow resistance remains finite, and flow cessation is not predicted at positive driving pressures. Nonetheless, the results suggest that the combined effects of elastic and viscous deformational resistance of red cells might lead to flow cessation at higher pressures than the estimates presented above, based on the elastic properties of the membrane. Studies to investigate this possibility are in progress.

Conclusions

Experimental observations of skeletal muscle show that recruitment of capillaries fed by a single arteriole can occur in a stepwise fashion. This implies that flow cessation can occur at small nonzero driving pressures in capillaries. Such behavior is not expected in uniform tubes, according to theoretical simulations. However, red cell motion may cease at nonzero driving pressures when red cells are unable to traverse irregular capillary geometries that they encounter. This behavior is likely to depend on both the elastic and the viscous components of resistance of the red cell membrane to transient deformation. Thus, the mechanical properties of red blood cells can play a significant role in determining functional capillary density.

Acknowledgement

This work was supported by NIH grants HL34555, HL17421 and HL07249.

References

1 Krogh A: The supply of oxygen to the tissues and the regulation of the capillary circulation. J Physiol 1919;52:457–474.
2 Ragan DMS, Schmidt EE, MacDonald IC, Groom AC: Spontaneous cyclic contractions of the capillary wall in vivo impeding red-cell flow: A quantitative analysis. Evidence for endothelial contractility. Microvasc Res 1988;36: 13–30.
3 Honig CR, Odoroff CL, Frierson JL: Capillary recruitment in exercise: Rate, extent, uniformity and relation to blood flow. Am J Physiol 1980;238:H31–H42.
4 Duling BR, Damon DH: An examination of the measurement of flow heterogeneity in striated muscle. Circ Res 1987;60:1–13.
5 Lund N, Damon DH, Damon DN, Duling BR: Capillary grouping in hamster tibialis anterior muscles: Flow patterns, and physiological significance. Int J Microcirc Clin Exp 1987;5: 359–372.
6 Lindbom L, Arfors KE: Mechanisms and site of control for variation in the number of perfused capillaries in skeletal muscle. Int J Microcirc Clin Exp 1985;4:19–30.
7 Delashaw JB, Duling BR: A study of the functional elements regulating capillary perfusion in striated muscle. Microvasc Res 1988;36: 162–171.
8 Skalak R: Rheology of red blood cell membrane; in Grayson J, Zingg W (eds): Microcirculation. New York, Plenum, 1976, vol 1, pp 53–70.
9 Hochmuth RM, Waugh RE: Erythrocyte membrane elasticity and viscosity. Annu Rev Physiology 1987;49:209–219.
10 Evans EA: Bending elastic modulus of red blood cell membrane derived from buckling instability in micropipet aspiration tests. Biophys J 1983;43:27–30.
11 Evans EA, Hochmuth RM: Membrane viscoelasticity. Biophys J 1976;16:1–11.
12 Canham PB, Burton AC: Distribution of size and shape in populations of normal human red blood cells. Circ Res 1968;22:405–422.
13 Halpern D, Secomb TW: The squeezing of red blood cells through capillaries with near-minimal diameters. J Fluid Mech 1989;203:381–400.
14 Meyer JU, Lindbom L, Intaglietta M: Coordinated diameter oscillations at arteriolar bifurcations in skeletal muscle. Am J Physiol 1987; 253:H568–H573.
15 Secomb TW, Skalak R, Özkaya N, Gross JF: Flow of axisymmetric red blood cells in narrow capillaries. J Fluid Mech 1986;163:405–423.
16 Secomb TW: Flow-dependent rheological properties of blood in capillaries. Microvasc Res 1987;34:46–58.
17 Secomb TW: Red blood cell mechanics and capillary blood rheology. Cell Biophysics 1991; 18:231–251.
18 Ellis CG, Tyml K, Strang BK: Variation in axial velocity profile of red cells passing through a single capillary; in Rakusan K, Biro GP, Goldstick TK, Turek Z (eds): Oxygen Transport to Tissue, X. New York, Plenum, 1989, pp 543–550.
19 Cokelet GR, Sarelius IH: Perceived vessel lumen and cell-blood velocity ratio: Impacts on in vivo blood flow rate determination. Am J Physiol 1992;262:H1156–H1163.
20 Secomb TW, Fleischman GJ, Papenfuss HD, Intaglietta M, Gross JF: Effects of reduced perfusion and hematocrit on flow distribution in capillary networks; in Messmer K, Hammersen F (eds): Microcirculation and Inflammation: Vessel Wall – Inflammatory Cells – Mediator Interaction. Prog Appl Microcirc. Basel, Karger, 1987, vol 12, pp 205–211.
21 Koller A, Johnson PC: Methods for in-vivo mapping and classifying vessel networks; in Popel AS, Johnson PC (eds): Microvascular Networks: Experimental and Theoretical Studies. Basel, Karger, 1986, pp 27–31.
22 Secomb TW, Gross JF: Flow of red blood cells in narrow capillaries: Role of membrane tension. Int J Microcirc Clin Exp 1983;2:229–240.
23 Secomb TW: Mechanics of blood flow in the microcirculation; in Ellington CP, Pedley TJ (eds): Biological Fluid Dynamics. London, Company of Biologists, in press.
24 Pries AR, Secomb TW, Gaehtgens P, Gross JF: Blood flow in microvascular networks – Experiments and simulation. Circ Res 1990;67:826–834.

Int J Microcirc 1995;15:255–264

G.W. Schmid-Schönbein
J. Lee

Department of Bioengineering and
Institute for Biomedical Engineering
University of California, San Diego
La Jolla, Calif., USA

Leukocytes in Capillary Flow

Key Words
Erythrocytes
Platelets
Endothelium
Aggregation
Adhesion
Capillary obstruction
Ischemia
Shock
Adhesion molecules

Abstract
During disease, the flow of blood cells through the capillary network is one of the most perilous events in the microcirculation. Capillary distensibility, cytoplasmic activity of endothelial cells, red cells and leukocytes play an important role in capillary perfusion. Occlusion of capillaries is one of the early signs of vascular failure and is encountered in many different conditions and organs. Adhesion of leukocytes to the endothelium via expression of membrane adhesion molecules leads to microvascular entrapment with capillary occlusion.

Introduction

One of the microcirculatory failures in the ischemic state and during reperfusion is the lack of unrestricted passage of blood cells through the microcirculation. The restriction of blood cell motion is in many situations first noted in the capillary network where blood cells need to pass in a single file. Restriction of blood cell motion in capillaries can take on different degrees of severity, and it finds its culmination in frank obstruction of the capillary network, even after restoration of the central perfusion pressure to control values. Dr. Guido Majno coined the term *no-reflow phenomenon* [1]. No-reflow in the capillary network can be observed in different organs in ischemia followed by reperfusion [2–5]. We will examine here some of the underlying mechanisms. Our discussion will be limited mostly to capillaries per se.

Capillary Distensibility and Lumen Shapes

Blood flow in capillaries has a low Reynolds number so that together with the pressure drop, viscous forces in the plasma dominate. One of the important consequences of this condition is that the shape of the lumen of blood vessels is an important determinant of flow. Nowhere in the circulation is a change of the endothelial cell shape more important than in capillaries, since they have the smallest lumen dimension compared with the size of the endothelial cells. Several morphological investigations have shown that the lumen cross sectional shape in arterioles changes during smooth muscle contraction [6, 7]. In capillaries, endothelial and lumen shape changes have been observed repeatedly [8–11], but few systematic investigations of the phenomenon have been completed. Noncircular lumen cross sections have important implications with respect to blood flow. For example, Poiseuille's formula has only limited application in noncircular cross sections; the ratio between maximum and mean velocity rises above the value of 2 in circular vessel cross sections so that cells in the center line can move faster than twice the mean velocity and the tube hematocrit may fall below val-

Dr. Geert W. Schmid-Schönbein
Department of Bioengineering
University of California, San Diego
La Jolla, CA 92093-0412 (USA)

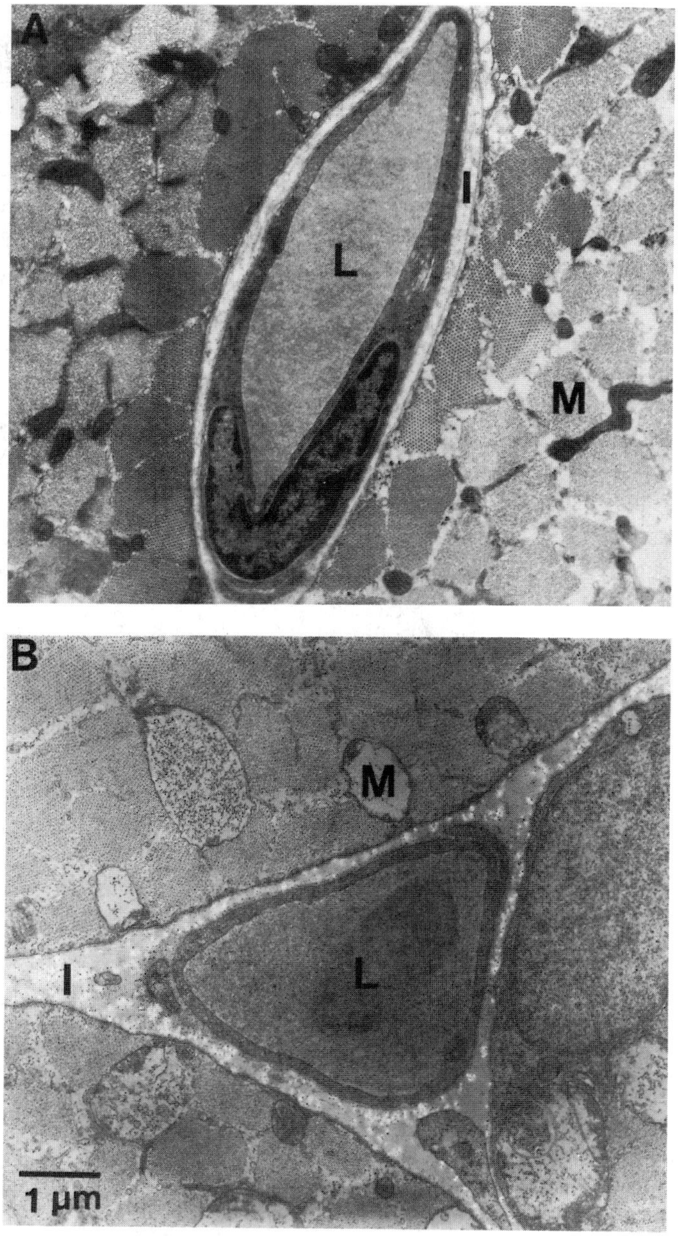

Fig. 1. Capillary cross sections in rat gracilis muscle (M) after fixation with 25 cm H_2O intravascular pressure. The section was cut at close to 90° to the long axis of the capillary. A capillary cross section is shown (**A**) positioned between two skeletal muscle fibers with elongated elliptical lumen cross section (L). A capillary in the junction between three muscle fibers (**B**) has a triangular cross section. The interstitial space (I) is small so that the skeletal muscle fibers (M) have a significant influence on the capillary lumen shape. Adopted from Lee and Schmid-Schönbein [18]. See this reference for methods.

ues in circular cylindrical capillaries, and the wall shear stress on the endothelium becomes highly nonuniform.

Directly related to the question of lumen shape is capillary distensibility. The blood stream is driven by a pressure gradient. Since the capillary lumen is distended by the local pressure, the resistance is a function of pressure. Thus the pressure distribution depends on the flow which in turn depends on the blood vessel distention. Several studies in different peripheral tissues have confirmed that capillaries are distensible [12–17]. They exhibit nonlinear pressure-diameter curves and viscoelastic features, such as creep or relaxation. In muscle capillary, the cross section is generally noncircular (fig.,1). Furthermore at low transmural pressures, the capillary lumen shapes are significantly distorted [18]. In skeletal muscle, the distortion is caused by compression of skeletal muscle fibers surrounding the capillary and/or by deformation of the endothelial cells. The distortion of the vessel lumen may reach the point where only a thin slit remains of the lumen (fig. 2), too narrow for either erythrocytes or leukocytes to pass. Relaxation of the endothelial cells during reduction of the transmural pressure can be accompanied by incorporation of plasma membrane and formation of cytoplasmic plasmalemmal vesicles which results in an apparent increase in the endothelial cytoplasmic volume. In contrast, elevation of the transmural pressure causes stretching of the endothelial cells (fig. 3), rounding of the capillary lumen and unfolding of plasmalemmal vesicles (fig. 4), an increase of the cell surface perimeter at both the luminal and abluminal side, and a reduction of the endothelial volume. The phenomenon may contribute to the apparent swelling of the endothelial cells observed in vivo [20], which is discussed more in detail by Mazzoni et al. in this issue. The distortion of the capillary lumen at reduced arterial pressures is accompanied by a significant rise in the hemodynamic resistance [18].

In addition to the passive deformation of endothelial cells under different transmural pressures, there is also experimental evidence to suggest that endothelial cells can project pseudopods, expecially during reduced transmural pressures [8, 21, 22]. Frequently, these projections originate at cell junctions and are pointing into the lumen (fig. 5). In skeletal muscle, pseudopods tend to project in sheet-like shapes, are organelle free, and appear to be made up largely of F-actin, rendering these structures relatively rigid [18]. The cytoplasmic projections grow predominantly into the lumen, with fewer projections into the basement membrane. Depending on the number and size, endothelial pseudopods strongly influence the capillary hemodynamic resistance [18].

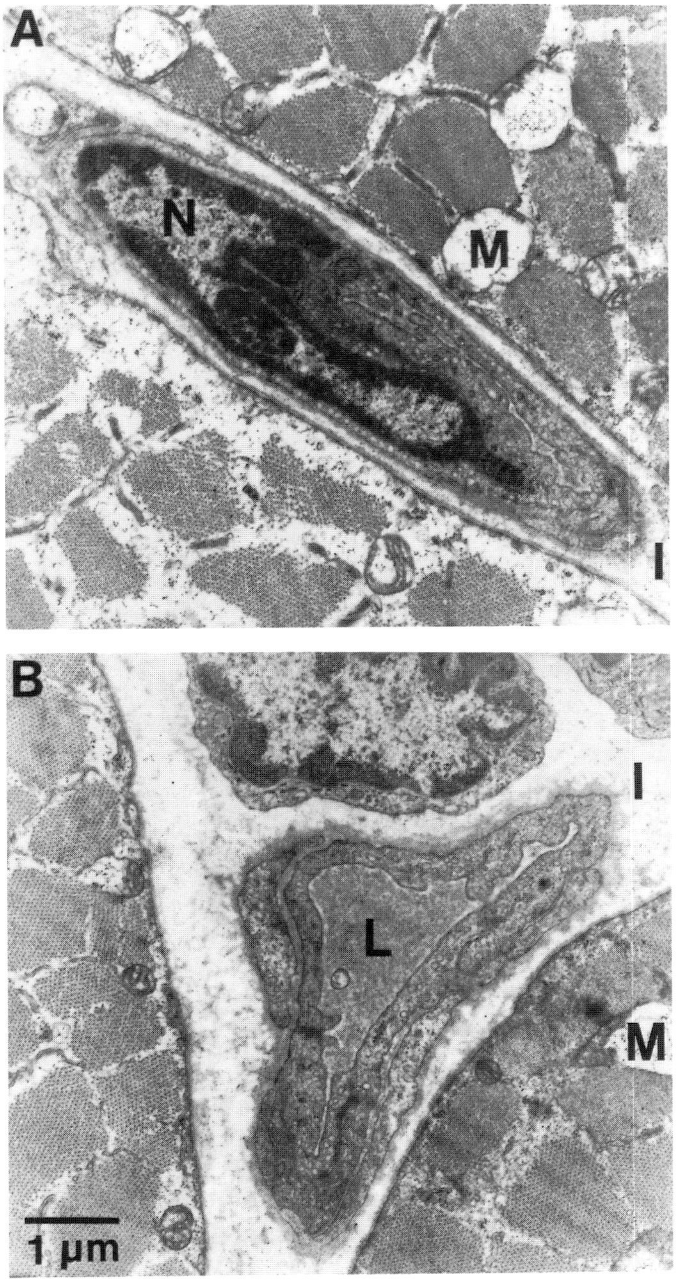

Fig. 2. Capillary cross sections in rat gracilis muscle after fixation with 0 cm H_2O intravascular pressure. The use of symbols is the same as in figure 1. Note that the capillary lumen is reduced to a single slit and the nucleus (N) is in part rounded. Adopted from Lee and Schmid-Schönbein [18].

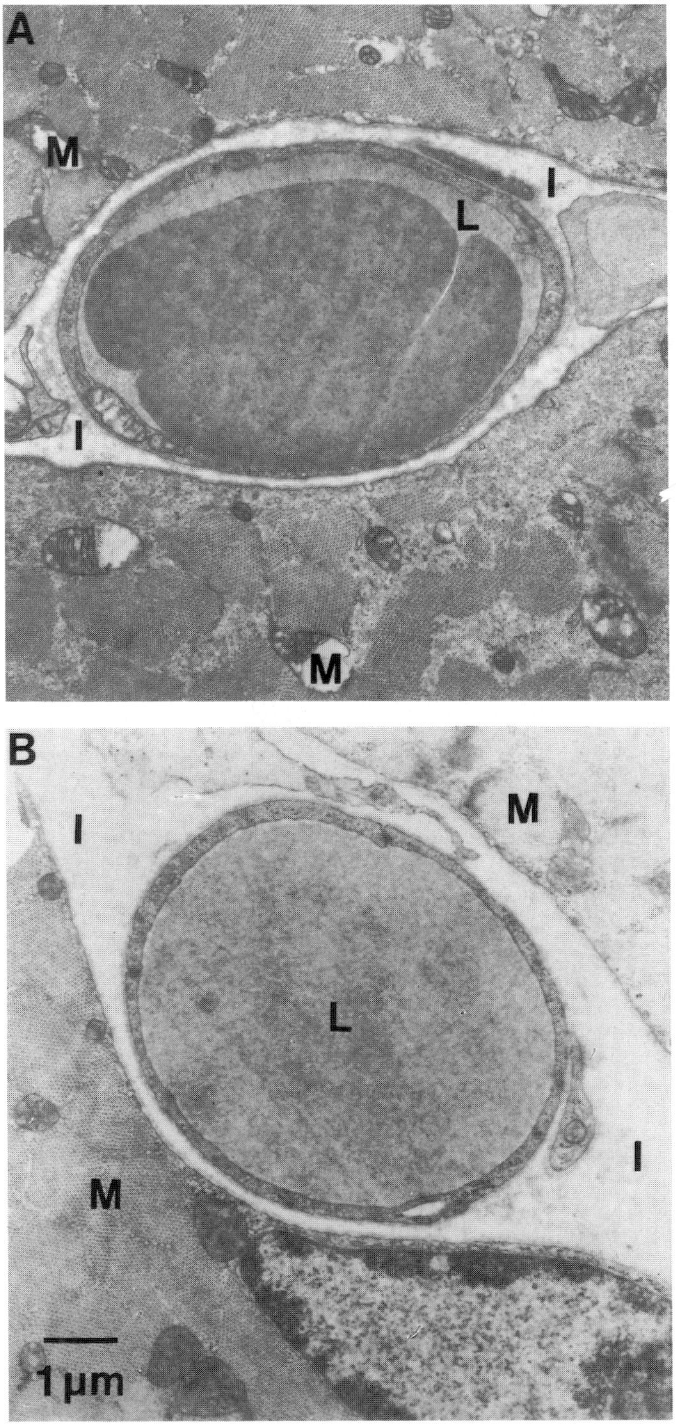

Fig. 3. Capillary cross sections in rat gracilis muscle after fixation with 50 cm H_2O intravascular pressure. The use of symbols is the same as in figure 1. Note that the capillary lumens are distended to almost circular cross sections and the endothelium is stretched. Adopted from Lee and Schmid-Schönbein [18].

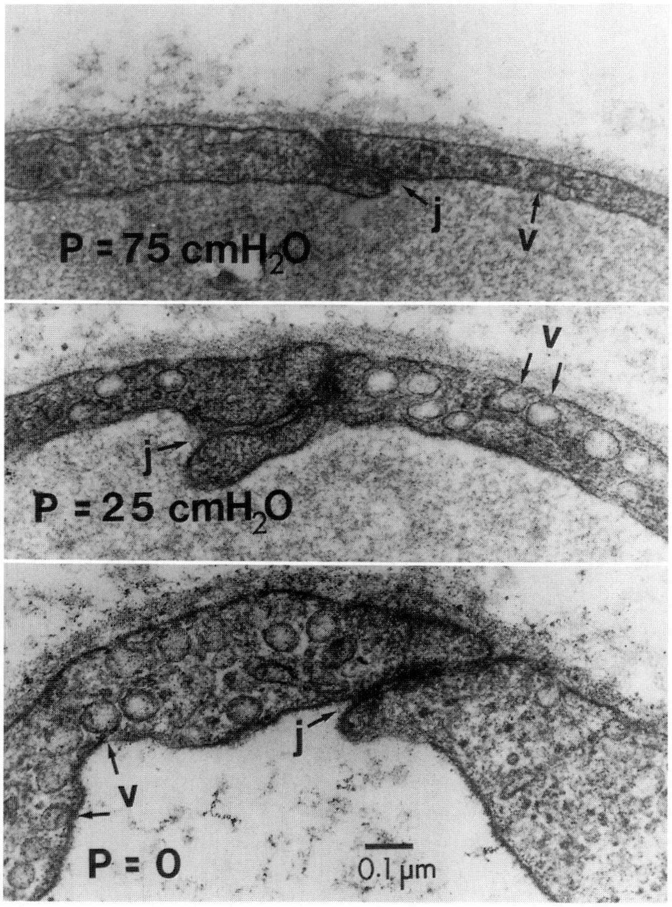

Fig. 4. Cross sections of capillary endothelium in rat gracilis muscle at different transmural pressures. Sections close to the endothelial junctions (j) are shown. Note the reduction and loss of plasmalemmal vesicles (v) as the endothelial cells become stretched with increasing transmural pressures (P). From Lee [19].

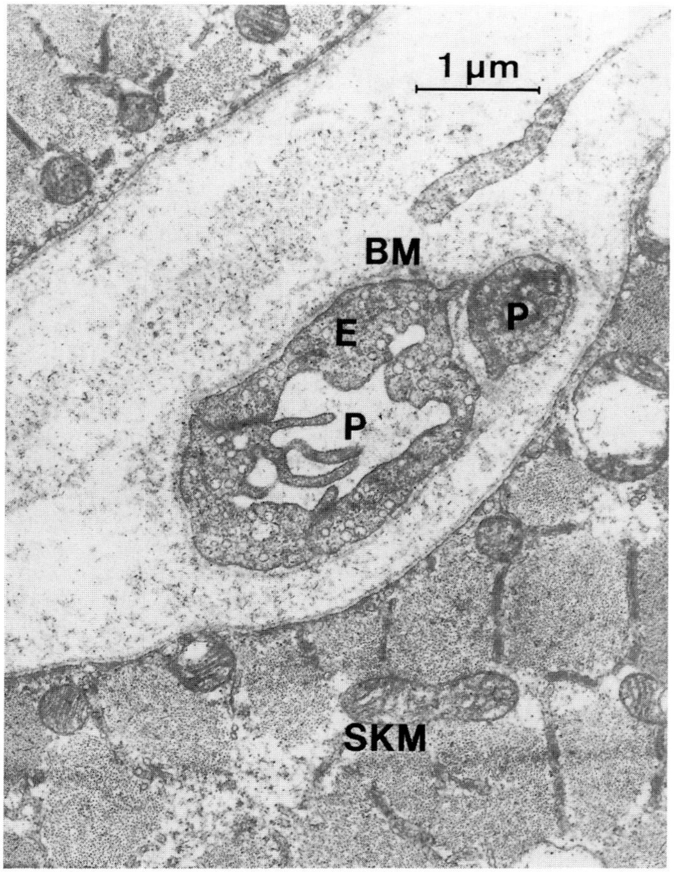

Fig. 5. Capillary cross sections in rat skeletal muscle (SKM) at zero capillary pressure after perfusion with an albumin-free buffer. The pressure was maintained for 10 min and then the capillary was fixed with an isotonic, pH-balanced, glutaraldehyde fixative in the same way as in figures 1–3. Prominent pseudopods (P) are projecting from the endothelial cell (E) into the lumen but not towards the basement membrane (BM). Similar pseudopods are encountered after stimulation with f-Met-Leu-Phe at low transmural pressures. From Lee [19].

Capillary Entry

In the majority of organs, both erythrocytes and leukocytes need to deform in order to pass through the capillary network. Platelets require less deformation due to their small size. The deformation takes place initially at the tapered entry into a capillary (fig. 6A). In the tapered entry region, erythrocytes and leukocytes are compressed by the pressure in the plasma fluid gap between the blood cell and the endothelial membrane. If the entry time is slow, the thickness of the fluid gap between the blood cell and endothelium may be small so that the outer glycocalyces on each membrane may slide over each other. This situation may be especially relevant with respect to circulating leukocytes since they are less deformable than erythrocytes and have plasma membrane folds which favor penetration of the fluid gap and close membrane contact. The highly flexible erythrocytes are rapidly deformed even if pulled into relatively narrow capillaries [23]. In contrast, the capillary entry time for the stiffer leukocytes is significantly longer [24–27].

Leukocytes are deformed into elongated shapes during viscoelastic creep [28–30], a process which is sensitive with respect to the pressure drop across the cell and to its cytoplasmic properties. The entry time into a capillary depends nonlinearly on the capillary diameter. An estimate of the entry time, t_E, for human neutrophils was derived from micropipette aspiration experiments [30] in the form

$$t_E = \frac{4}{3}\frac{\eta}{\Delta P}\left\{\left(\frac{r_c}{a}\right)^3 - \left[1+\ln\left(\frac{r_c}{a}\right)^3\right]\right\},$$

where r_c is the undeformed cell radius, a is the capillary radius, η is the cytoplasmic viscosity during the continuous deformation phase of the neutrophil, and ΔP is the pressure drop across the neutrophil. It is apparent from this relationship, that the entry time is strongly dependent on the diameter a of the capillary, so that even fractions of one micrometer may significantly influence the movement of leukocytes. The larger monocytes and granulocytes require a longer entry time than the smaller lymphocytes.

The velocity of leukocytes in arterioles is rapidly reduced at the entry into the capillaries and the deformation phase is accompanied by a slow forward velocity [23]. Under intravital conditions, this has been referred to as *temporary plugging* at the entry into capillaries [31, 32]. Typical times for temporary plugging of neutrophils and monocytes in skeletal muscle are about 100 ms to 1 s [31, 33] and depend on the cytoskeletal properties of the leukocytes [33, 34]. Entry times for red cells are significantly shorter, of the order of 5–10 ms.

The degree of leukocyte deformation at the entry to capillaries depends on the presence of smooth muscle constriction at the terminal endings of small arterioles (fig. 6B). Such structures consist of a terminal coil of smooth muscle positioned largely at the capillary entry region and have been referred to in the past as capillary sphincters. Partial constriction of smooth muscle causes local narrowing of the capillary lumen diameter at the entry to a value which is smaller than the diameter of the capillary per se. When leukocytes enter into such capillaries, their shape is compressed at the entry into a narrower dimension than necessary for passage through the capillary, providing an enlarged lubrication layer and rapid passage of leukocytes through the capillary. In contrast, in the low-flow state with reduced arterial pressures, the myogenic constrictor stimulus is reduced and the terminal arterioles are dilated. The local constriction at the entry into the capillary is no longer present, and leukocytes are deformed to a lesser degree. The reduced deformation of the leukocyte, reduced transmural pressure and recoil of the capillary lumen, as well as reduced pressure drop along the length of the capillary set up a situation where leukocytes may no longer be able to pass through the lumen.

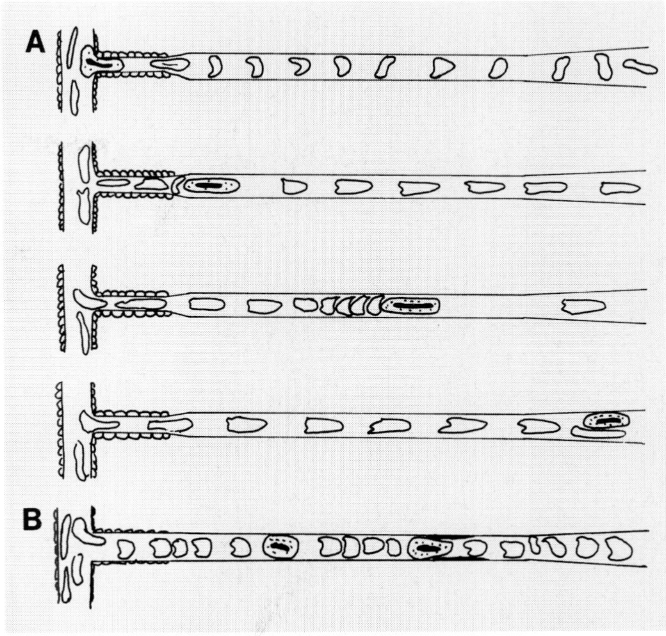

Fig. 6. Schematic of leukocyte entry into and passage through a capillary. **A** Entry (first sketch), and rapid passage of a leukocyte (second sketch) with train formation (third sketch) and systematic attachment to postcapillary endothelium (fourth sketch). The leukocyte is compressed upon entry at the capillary sphincter to a dimension that is narrower than required for free passage through the remainder of the capillary. **B** In the low-flow state, with reduced myogenic response, the terminal smooth muscle is dilated and leukocytes are no longer deformed to the same degree. During passage through the capillary, leukocytes are less deformed and interact more strongly with the endothelium, especially if endothelial cells relax passively due to the pressure reduction (not shown). Leukocyte capillary obstruction may occur.

Capillary Entrapment of Blood Cells

Red cell aggregate formation, platelet aggregate formation and leukocyte plugging are mechanisms for capillary obstruction. Under experimental conditions, red cell aggregates are relatively weak. While they may form under low-flow conditions, they are readily swept out of the capillary network if the perfusion pressure is restored to normal physiological values [35]. There is currently little experimental evidence from acute experiments to suggest that platelet aggregates participate in capillary obstruction. Chronic conditions are, however, largely unexplored in this respect.

The high cellular stiffness and ability of leukocytes to adhere to the endothelium are significant risk factors for capillary obstruction. One of the conditions under which

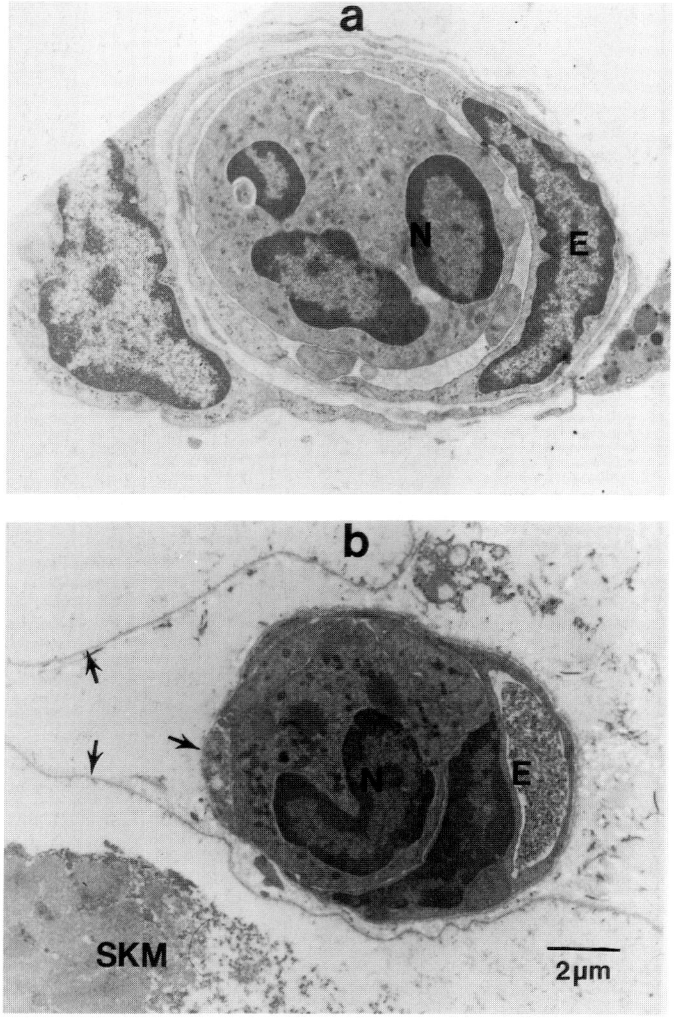

Fig. 7. Transmission electron micrograph of neutrophil (N) capillary obstruction in rat spinotrapezius muscle (SKM) after a low-flow period for 1 h (**a**) and 4 h (**b**) at 40 mm Hg mean central blood pressure followed by reperfusion for 15 min at normal blood pressure. There is initially no indication of significant swelling of the endothelial cell cytoplasm (E), although after prolonged ischemia significant deformation of the endothelial cells can be demonstrated with open junctions and detachment of basement membrane (arrows) from the muscle cells. From Schmid-Schönbein [37].

circulating leukocytes may become entrapped in capillaries is by reduction of the arterial pressure [36]. The requirements for neutrophils to remain *stationary* in capillaries in the presence of a perfusion pressure is by adhesion to the endothelium (fig. 7). Adhesion to the capillary endothelium may reach different levels depending on the nature of the adhesion mechanisms involved and the formation of a membrane contact region. It may reach such high levels of membrane adhesion energy, that leukocytes will withstand normal physiological perfusion pressure and obstruct capillary regions. Capillary no-reflow is encountered in many different organs [3, 38–44]. Immunoprotection of leukocyte membrane integrins (CD18) with monoclonal antibodies serves to reduce the membrane adhesion stress and abolish the capillary non-reflow [45, 46]. After acute ischemia and reperfusion, occluded capillaries are intact, there is mild if any swelling of the endothelium or death of endothelial cells [47], and packed red cells and occasional platelets are observed. Neutrophils in the capillaries are deformed into cylindrical shapes with close membrane abutment to the endothelium (fig. 7).

Accumulations of leukocytes in the microcirculation can also be observed in hemorrhagic or endotoxic shock [2, 48]. In these situations, virtually all organs are affected, and the entrapment of circulating leukocytes in microvessels occurs early after pressure reduction or endotoxin administration, respectively. The reasons for this initial leukocyte trapping in hemorrhagic versus endotoxic shock are, however, different. In hemorrhagic shock it is due to the pressure reduction, in endotoxic shock it is due to activation of the leukocytes and endothelium with enhancement of the membrane adhesion and with pseudopod formation.

Neutropenia [2, 41, 42, 49–52] or immunoprotection of adhesion proteins [46, 53–57] have been shown to be beneficial in many models of ischemia and in hemorrhagic shock. Obstructed capillaries also contain many red cells and platelets, but both cell types are passively trapped due to the leukocyte obstruction [58]. At the moment when the leukocyte is pushed out of an obstructed capillary, all red cells and platelets are washed out of the capillary and flow is restored [36, 59].

Entrapment of leukocytes in the microcirculation promotes capillary no-reflow and interrupts nutrient and metabolite transport to the tissue. At the same time, it leads to a global immunological suppression, since entrapped leukocytes have a reduced likelihood of contact with microorganisms to carry out phagocytosis. Attachment of leukocytes to the postcapillary endothelium is associated with oxygen free radical formation, especially in gap region between leukocytes and endothelial membranes [60]. Free radical formation involves membrane attachment via the integrins (CD11b/CD18) [61]. In the absence of antithrombotic agents, leukocytes also serve platelet aggregate formation with adhesion to the endothelium and fibrin deposition [3, 39]. The presence of leukocytes in platelet thrombi is mediated by P-selectin [62].

Leukocyte Capillary Obstructions in Chronic Conditions

In contrast to the acute occlusions, the capillary obstructions under chronic conditions, such as diabetic retinopathy, are almost exclusively due to monocyte entrapment in the capillary network [63]. Vascular lesions occur exclusively in regions of monocyte accumulation, even after a prolonged diabetic state. Accumulation of the monocytes is accompanied by injury to the endothelium and interstitial cells and phagocytosis by monocytes/macrophages. The cause for the enhanced trapping of monocytes in the microcirculation of diabetics appears to be induction of spontaneous monocyte activation, since there is no apparent compromise of the central blood pressure. The spontaneous activation of the circulating neutrophils and monocytes correlates closely with elevation of the blood glucose level, even at early stages after initiation of the diabetic state.

Parenchymal Cell Death

What are the consequences of low flow or obstruction of capillaries for cell viability? Besides the interruption of the oxygen supply and metabolite removal, there is evidence that oxygen free radicals may be formed. Cell death in ischemia/reperfusion and inflammation appear to be caused by different mechanisms. Observation of leukocytes and platelet motion in conjunction with markers for cell death by digital fluorescent microscopy has revealed a sequence of events that leads to the actual death of parenchymal cells. During ischemia in rat skeletal muscle, leukocytes are trapped in capillaries and postcapillary venules, while minimal cell death occurs. Instead, the major cell death occurs during early reperfusion even at a time when the majority of leukocytes and platelets that have accumulated during ischemia are washed out of the muscle microcirculation. Cell death is restricted to parenchymal fibers that have limited antioxidative capacity. Cell death during initial reperfusion is mediated in part by the endothelial cells of reperfused capillaries and can be attenuated with a xanthine oxidase inhibitor. Neutrophils are not involved in the initial cell death [47]. Instead, neutrophils become trapped after reperfusion when normal pressures have been restored with capillary occlusion as well as adhesion to postcapillary venules. About one hour after reperfusion, there is again increased accumulation of granulocytes in the microcirculation with recurrence of capillary obstruction, adhesion to postcapillaries, interstitial migration and extensive parenchymal cell death. The release of free radicals upon reperfusion sets into motion a number of intracellular responses from programmed cell death, initiation of gene expression, degranulation, nitric oxide and superoxide production, and necrosis.

Cell Activation and Interventions

There are two principal pathways for leukocyte and platelet trapping in the microcirculation in the low-flow state. Either preactivated cells in the active circulation become trapped in the microcirculation, or nonactivated cells adhere to activated endothelium in the microcirculation and then in turn become activated, as in a classical inflammatory response. Combinations of the two processes may occur frequently. The sequence of events will differ from case to case and is important to identify for designing new interventions. An array of substances and products activates leukocytes, peptide sequences (f-Met-Leu-Phe and analogs), complement products, leukotrienes, cytokines, platelet-activating factor, endotoxins, tissue breakdown products, thrombotic products, oxidized products and others. Activation of neutrophils is manifest in the form of pseudopod formation (fig. 8), free radical production, expression of adhesion proteins, and degranulation. Each of these forms of activation may contribute to microvascular entrapment and organ injury.

The mechanism of cell activation in ischemia and reperfusion is less certain at the moment, since in these situations no activator is added either centrally into the blood stream or locally in the tissue. There is evidence that platelet activating factor and leukotrienes may be released [65, 66]. In contrast, in endotoxic shock the initial activator that triggers cell activation is administered into the circulation. Endotoxin stimulates endothelial dysfunction, and platelet and leukocyte activation by several pathways including the endotoxin-binding mechanism, tumor necrosis factor formation, expression of adhesion proteins, microvascular entrapment of circulating leukocytes, and parenchymal cell death [67].

Low activation is accompanied by decreased frequency of leukocyte capillary entrapment. An example is endotoxin-tolerant animals after both endotoxic or hemorrhagic shock [68]. Following the cardiovascular challenge, tolerant animals have low levels of cell activation in the circulation and exhibit reduced microvascular entrapment of leukocytes with less capillary occlusion and improved survival rates.

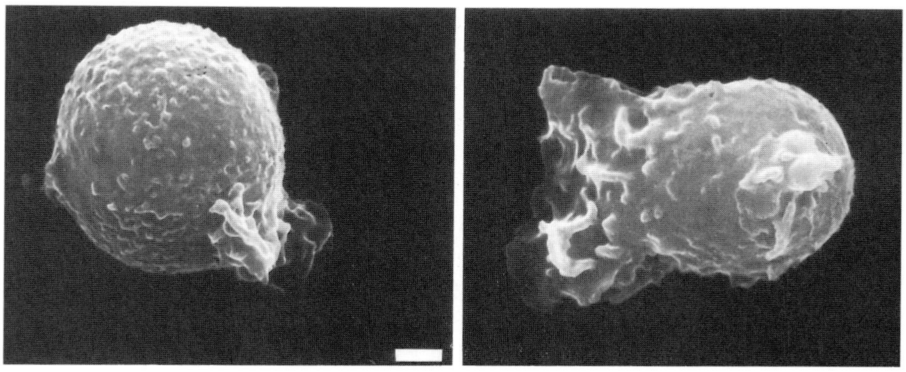

Fig. 8. Scanning electron micrograph of human leukocytes with small (left) and larger (right) active cytoplasmic pseudopods. The cells were fixed in free suspension and dehydrated by critical-point drying, as described previously [64]. Pseudopods consist of rigidified actin with localized expression of adhesion proteins which leads to an enhanced probability for microvascular trapping of leukocytes. Cells with larger pseudopods encounter significantly higher probability for microvascular entrapment. Bar = 1 μm.

Initiation of Leukocyte Attachment to Postcapillary Endothelium

The initial events that lead to leukocyte attachment to postcapillary endothelium have their origin in the capillaries. Inside a capillary, leukocytes move with lower velocity than erythrocytes [69]. This difference in velocity is sufficient to lead to characteristic leukocyte-erythrocyte train formation inside capillaries. Due to hydrodynamic interaction, the erythrocytes displace the leukocytes from their central position in the lumen of a capillary towards an off-center position closer to the endothelium. At the point where the lumen of the capillary widens, such that the leukocyte can rotate, red cells tend to pass the slower-moving leukocytes. During passage, the erythrocytes displace the leukocytes from a central position in the capillary lumen towards the wall of the postcapillary venules so that membrane attachment between leukocyte and endothelium is possible. Each leukocyte passing through the microcirculation is pushed close to the endothelium and thereby initiates the membrane adhesion process. The interaction requires the erythrocytes, since under experimental conditions, when erythrocytes are removed from the circulation, few leukocytes become attached to the endothelium and most leukocytes that enter the microcirculation on the arteriolar side exit on the venular side [70]. Systematic membrane contact between leukocytes and endothelium is also initiated at convergent bifurcations of postcapillary venules [71].

Capillary Resistance

In addition to the shape changes of capillary endothelium under different pressures, the passage of red cells and also circulating leukocytes may significantly elevate the hemodynamic resistance in capillaries. The additional pressure drop imposed by a single leukocyte in rat gracilis muscle with dilated arterioles and without significant adhesion to the endothelium is about three orders of magnitude larger than the additional pressure drop of one erythrocyte [72]. Activation of leukocytes leads to further elevation of the additional pressure drop of leukocytes. While this large pressure drop may in part be due to a narrow lubrication layer of leukocytes in capillaries [73], the temporary plugging at the entry to capillaries causes a transient very low velocity inside the capillary and thus high resistance. If such instances of high resistance occur frequently at different locations of the capillary network, the average organ resistance, as measured at the inflow arteries, increases. Under normal conditions, leukocytes flow along preferential pathways in the distal portion of the microcirculation. For significant increase in organ resistance to occur, the leukocyte pathways need to be distributed throughout the capillary network [32]. Another mechanism that may contribute to the elevation of capillary resistance in the presence of leukocytes is disturbance of red cell motion. Erythrocytes positioned upstream of a leukocyte in a single file capillary are subject to tumbling with frequent change of shape, rotation and disturbance of the lubrication layer. This serves to elevate the hemodynamic resistance in the capillary [74].

Conclusion

No other part of the circulation is as susceptible to vascular failure as the capillary network. It is the segment where blood cells are subject to the greatest deformation in the circulation and where strong interactions exist with the endothelium for each and every cell in the circulation. A shift in endothelial cell shape, a change in cytoplasmic mechanical properties or membrane adhesion will raise the pressure drop required for individual blood cells to pass the capillary network. Individual capillaries and segments of the capillary network can trap blood cells with relative ease. A mild pressure reduction, activation of endothelial cells or leukocytes, or aggregation of platelets is sufficient to occlude capillaries. No aggregation of leukocytes is necessary. Leukocyte capillary plugging serves as a microvascular trapping mechanism for circulating leukocytes. The implications of capillary occlusion for cardiovascular disease and aging in humans remain to be explored in the future.

Acknowledgments

This work was supported by the National Institutes of Health Program Project Grant HL-43026 (Director Dr. Shu Chien) and grant HL-10881.

References

1 Ames A, Wright R, Kowada M, Thurston JM, Majno G: Cerebral ischemia. II: The no-reflow phenomenon. Am J Pathol 1968;52:437–453.
2 Barroso-Aranda J, Schmid-Schönbein GW, Zweifach BW, Engler RL: Granulocytes and no-reflow phenomenon in irreversible hemorrhagic shock. Circ Res 1988;63:437–447.
3 Del Zoppo GJ, Schmid-Schönbein GW, Mori E, Copeland BR, Chang CM: Polymorphonuclear leukocytes occlude capillaries following middle cerebral artery occlusion and reperfusion. Stroke 1991;22:1276–1283.
4 Kloner RA, Ganote CE, Jennings RB: The 'no-reflow' phenomenon after temporary coronary occlusion in the dog. J Clin Invest 1974;54:1496–1508.
5 Korthuis RJ, Grisham MB, Granger DN: Leukocyte depletion attenuates vascular injury in postischemic skeletal muscle. Am J Physiol 1988;254:H823–H827.
6 Schmid-Schönbein GW, Murakami H: Blood flow in contracting arterioles. Int J Microcirc Clin Exp 1985;4:311–328.
7 Walmersley JG, Gore RW, Dacey RAJ, Damon DN, Duling BR: Quantitative morphology of arterioles from the hamster cheek pouch related to mechanical analysis. Microvasc Res 1982;24:249–271.
8 Gidlöf A, Lewis DH, Hammersen F: The effect of prolonged total ischemia on the ultrastructure of human skeletal muscle capillaries: A morphometric analysis. Int J Microcirc Clin Exp 1987;7:67–86.
9 Gidlöf A, Lewis DH, Hammersen F: Fine structure of the human skeletal muscle capillary: A morphometric analysis. Int J Microcirc Clin Exp 1987;7:43–66.
10 Hammersen F, Hammersen E: The ultrastructure of endothelial gap-formation and leukocyte emigration; in Messmer K, Hammersen F (eds): Microcirculation and Inflammation: Vessel Wall – Inflammatory Cells – Mediator Interaction. Prog Appl Microcirc. Basel, Karger, 1987, vol 12, pp 1–34.
11 Potter RF, Groom AC: Capillary diameter and geometry in cardiac and skeletal muscle studies by means of corrosion casts. Microvasc Res 1983;25:68–84.
12 Baez S, Lamport H, Baez A: Pressure effects in living microscopic vessels; in Copley AL, Stainsby G: Flow Properties of Blood. London, Pergamon, 1960, pp 122–136.
13 Baldwin AL, Gore RW: Simultaneous measurement of capillary distensibility and hydraulic conductance. Microvasc Res 1989;38:1–22.
14 Bouskela E, Wiederhielm C: Viscoelastic properties of capillaries. Microvasc Res 1979;17:S1.
15 Skalak TC, Schmid-Schönbein GW: Viscoelastic properties of microvessels in rat spinotrapezius muscle. J Biomech Eng 1986;108:193–200.
16 Smaje LH, Fraser PA, Clough G: The distensibility of single capillaries and venules in the cat mesentery. Microvasc Res 1980;20:358–370.
17 Swayne GTG, Smaje LH, Bergel DH: Distensibility of single capillaries and venules in the rat and frog mesentery. Int J Microcirc Clin Exp 1989;8:25–42.
18 Lee J, Schmid-Schönbein GW: Biomechanics of skeletal muscle capillaries: Hemodynamic resistance, endothelial distensibility, and pseudopod formation. Ann Biomed Eng 1995, in press.
19 Lee J: The Morphometry and Mechanical Properties of Skeletal Muscle Capillaries; PhD thesis University of California, 1990.
20 Mazzoni MC, Borgström P, Intaglietta M, Arfors KE: Lumenal narrowing and endothelial cell swelling in skeletal muscle capillaries during hemorrhagic shock. Circ Shock 1989;29:27–39.
21 Abbas B, Hume SP, McCullough JS, Wilson DJ, Stewart PC, Carr KE: Early morphological changes in blood capillaries of mouse duodenal villi induced by X-irradiation. J Submicrosc Cytol Pathol 1990;22:609–614.
22 Philpott DE, Popova IA, Kato K, Stevenson J, Miquel J, Sapp W: Morphological and biochemical examination of Cosmos 1887 rat heart tissue. Part I – Ultrastructure. FASEB J 1990;4:73–78.
23 Skalak R, Oskaya N, Skalak TC: Biofluid mechanics. Annu Rev Fluid Mech 1989;21:167–204.
24 Bagge U, Skalak R, Attefors R: Granulocyte rheology: Experimental studies in an in-vitro microflow system. Adv Microcirc 1972;7:29–48.
25 Fenton BM, Wilson DW, Cokelet GR: Analysis of the effects of measured white blood cell entrance times on hemodynamics in a computer model of a microvascular bed. Pflugers Arch 1985;403:395–401.
26 Warnke KC, Skalak TC: Leukocyte plugging in vivo in skeletal muscle arteriolar trees. Am J Physiol 1992;262:H1149–H1155.
27 Yamakawa T, Yamaguchi S, Sugiyama I: White blood cell plugging and blood flow maldistribution in the capillary network of cat cerebral cortex in acute hemorrhagic hypotension: An intravital microscopic study. Circ Shock 1987;22:323–332.
28 Dong C, Skalak R, Sung KLP: Cytoplasmic rheology of passive neutrophils. Biorheology 1991;28:557–568.
29 Dong C, Skalak R, Sung KLP, Schmid-Schönbein GW, Chien S: Passive deformation analysis of human leukocytes. J Biomech Eng 1988;110:27–36.
30 Needham D, Hochsmith RM: Rapid flow of passive neutrophils into a 4 μm pipet and measurement of cytoplasmic viscosity. J Biomech Eng 1990;112:269–276.
31 Gaehtgens P, Ley K, Pries AR, Müller R: Mutual interactions between leukocytes and microvascular blood flow; in Hammersen F, Messmer K (eds): White Cell Rheology and Inflammation. Prog Appl Microcirc. Basel, Karger, 1985, vol 7, pp 15–28.
32 Warnke KC, Skalak TC: The effects of leukocytes on blood flow in a model skeletal muscle capillary network. Microvasc Res 1990;40:118–136.
33 Harris AG, Skalak TC: Leukocyte cytoskeletal structure determines capillary plugging and network resistance. Am J Physiol 1993;265:H1670–H1675.
34 Worthen GS, Schwab B, Elson EL, Downey GP: Cellular mechanics of stimulated neutrophils: Stiffening of cells induces retention in pores in vitro and lung capillaries in vivo. Science 1989;245:183–186.

35 Driessen GK, Heidtmann H, Schmid-Schönbein H: Effect of hemodilution and hemoconcentration on red cell flow velocity in the capillaries of the rat mesentery. Pflügers Arch 1979; 380:1–6.
36 Bagge U: White blood cell deformability and plugging of skeletal muscle capillaries in hemorrhagic shock. Acta Physiol Scand 1980;108: 159–163.
37 Schmid-Schönbein GW: Granulocytes: Friend and foe. News Physiol Sci 1988;3:144–147.
38 Engler RL, Schmid-Schönbein GW, Pavelec RS: Leukocyte capillary plugging in myocardial ischemia and reperfusion in the dog. Am J Pathol 1983;111:98–111.
39 Garcia JH, Liu KF, Yishida Y, Lian J, Chen S, Del Zoppo GJ: The influx of leukocytes and platelets in an evolving brain infarct (Wistar rat). Am J Pathol 1994;144:188–199.
40 Hernandez L, Grisham M, Twohig B, Arfors K, Harlan J, Granger N: Role of neutrophils in ischemia reperfusion induced microvascular injury. Am J Physiol 1987;253:H699–H703.
41 Korthuis RJ, Grisham MB, Granger DN: Leukocyte depletion attenuates vascular injury in postischemic skeletal muscle. Am J Physiol 1988;254:H823–H827.
42 Smith SM, Holm-Rutili L, Perry MA, Grisham MB, Arfors KE, Granger DN, Kvietys PR: Role of neutrophils in hemorrhagic shock-induced gastric mucosal injury in the rat. Gastroenterology 1987;93:466–471.
43 Wilson JW: Leukocyte sequestration and morphologic augmentation in the pulmonary network following hemorrhagic shock and related forms of stress. Adv Microcirc 1972;4:197–232.
44 Yamakawa T, Sugiyama I, Hiimi H: Behavior of white blood cells in microcirculation of the cat brain cortex during hemorrhagic shock. Int J Microcirc Clin Exp 1984;3:554.
45 Jerome SN, Smith CW, Korthuis RJ: CD18-dependent adherence reactions play an important role in the development of the no-reflow phenomenon. J Appl Physiol 1993;264:H479–H483.
46 Mori E, Del Zoppo GJ, Chambers JD, Copeland BR, Arfors KE: Inhibition of polymorphonuclear leukocyte adherence suppresses no-reflow after focal cerebral ischemia in baboons. Stroke 1992;23:712–718.
47 Suematsu M, DeLano FA, Poole D, Engler RL, Miyasaka M, Zweifach BW, Schmid-Schönbein GW: Spatial and temporal correlation between leukocyte behavior and cell injury in postischemic rat skeletal muscle microcirculation. Lab Invest 1994;70:684–695.
48 Barroso-Aranda J, Schmid-Schönbein GW, Zweifach BW, Mathison JC: Polymorphonuclear neutrophil contribution to induced tolerance by bacterial lipopolysaccaride. Circ Res 1991;69:1196–1206.
49 Dutka AJ, Kochanek PM, Hallenbeck JM: Influence of granulocytopenia on canine cerebral ischemia induced by air embolism. Stroke 1989;20:390–395.
50 Engler RL, Dahlgren MD, Morris DD, Peterson MA, Schmid-Schönbein GW: Role of leukocytes in the response to acute myocardial ischemia and reflow in dogs. Am J Physiol 1986;251:H314–H322.
51 Romson JL, Hook BG, Kunkel SL, Abrams GD, Schork MA, Lucchesi BR: Reduction of the extent of ischemic myocardial injury by neutrophil depletion in the dog. Circulation 1983;67:1016–1023.
52 Vasthare US, Heinel LA, Rosenwasser RH, Tuma RF: Leukocyte involvement in cerebral ischemia and reperfusion injury. Surg Neurol 1990;33:261–265.
53 Ma XL, Tsao PS, Lefer AM: Antibody to CD-18 exerts endothelial and cardiac protective effects in myocardial ischemia and reperfusion. J Clin Invest 1991;88:1237–1243.
54 Ma XL, Lefer DJ, Lefer AM, Rothlein R: Coronary endothelial and cardiac protective effects of a monoclonal antibody to intercullular adhesion molecule-1 in myocardial ischemia and reperfusion. Circulation 1992;86:937–946.
55 Ma XL, Weyrich AS, Lefer DJ, Buerke M, Albertine KH, Kishimoto TK, Lefer AM: Monoclonal antibody to L-selectin attenuates neutrophil accumulation and protects ischemic reperfused cat myocardium. Circulation 1993; 88:649–658.
56 Simpson P, Todd R, Fantoen J, Mickelson J, Griffin J, Lucchesi B: Reduction of experimental canine myocardial reperfusion injury by a monoclonal antibody that inhibits leukocyte adhesion. J Clin Invest 1988;81:624–629.
57 Vedder N, Winn C, Rice C, Chi E, Arfors K, Harlan J: A monoclonal antibody to the adherence promoting leukocyte glycoprotein CD18, reduces organ injury and improves survival from hemorrhagic shock and resuscitation in rabbits. J Clin Invest 1988;81:939–944.
58 Mullane KM, Salmon JA, Kraemer R: Leukocyte derived metabolites of arachidonic acid in ischemia-induced myocardial injury. Fed Proc 1987;46:2422–2433.
59 Schmid-Schönbein GW: Mechanisms of granulocyte-capillary-plugging; in Messmer K, Hammersen F (eds): Microcirculation and Inflammation: Vessel Wall – Inflammatory Cells – Mediator Interaction. Prog Appl Microcirc. Basel, Karger, 1987, vol 12, pp 223–230.
60 Suematsu M, Kurose I, Asako H, Miura S, Tsuchiya M: In-vivo visualization of oxyradical-dependent photo emission during endothelium-granulocyte interaction in microvascular beds treated with platelet-activating factor. J Biochem 1989;106:355–360.
61 Suematsu M, Schmid-Schönbein GW, Chávez-Chávez RH, Yee TT, Tamatami T, Miyasaka M, DeLano FA, Zweifach BW: In vivo visualization of oxidative changes in microvessels during neutrophil activation. Am J Physiol 1993;264:H881–H891.
62 Palabrica T, Lobb R, Furie BC, Aronovitz M, Benjamin C, Hsu YM, Sajer SA, Furie B: Leukocyte accumulation promoting fibrin deposition is mediated in vivo by P-selectin on adherent platelets. Nature 1992;359:848–851.
63 Schröder S, Palinski W, Schmid-Schönbein GW: Activated monocytes and granulocytes, capillary non-perfusion and neovascularization in diabetic retinopathy. Am J Pathol 1991;139: 81–100.
64 Schmid-Schönbein GW, Shih YY, Chien S: Morphometry of human leukocytes. Blood 1980;56:866–875.
65 Lehr HA, Guhlman A, Nolte D, Keppler D, Messmer K: Leukotrienes as mediators in ischemia-reperfusion injury in a microcirculation model in the hamster. J Clin Invest 1991;87: 2036–2041.
66 Mozes T, Braquet P, Filip J: Platelet-activating factor: An endogenous mediator of mesenteric ischemia-reperfusion induced shock. Am J Physiol 1989;257:R872–R877.
67 Barroso-Aranda J, Schmid-Schönbein GW: Transformation of neutrophils as indicator of irreversibility in hemorrhagic shock. Am J Physiol 1989;257:H846–H852.
68 Barroso-Aranda J, Chavez-Chavez R, Mathison JC, Suematsu M, Schmid-Schönbein GW: Circulating neutrophil kinetics during tolerance in hemorrhagic schock using bacterial lipopolysaccharide. Am J Physiol 1994;266: H415–H421.
69 Mayrovitz HN: The relationship between leukocytes and erythrocytes velocity in arterioles; in Bagge U, Born GVR, Gaehtgens P (eds): White Blood Cells, Morphology and Rheology as Related to Function. The Hague, Martinus Nijhoff, 1982, pp 82–88.
70 Bagge U, Blixt A, Strid KG: The initiation of post-capillary margination of leukocytes: Studies in vitro on the influence of erythrocyte concentration and flow velocity. Int J Microcirc Clin Exp 1983;2:215–227.
71 Bagge U, Karlsson R: Maintenance of white cell margination at the passage through small venular junctions. Microvasc Res 1980;20:92–95.
72 Sutton DW, Schmid-Schönbein GW: Elevation of organ resistance due to leukocyte perfusion. Am J Physiol 1992;262:H1646–H1650.
73 Schmid-Schönbein GW, Skalak R, Usami S, Chien S: Cell distribution in capillary networks. Microvasc Res 1980;19:18–44.
74 Thompson TN, La Celle PL, Cokelet GR: Perturbation of red cell flow in small tubes by white blood cells. Pflügers Arch 1989;413:372–377.

Int J Microcirc 1995;15:265–270

Michelle C. Mazzoni
P. Borgström
K.C. Warnke
T.C. Skalak
M. Intaglietta
K.E. Arfors

Institute for Biomedical Engineering,
University of California, San Diego,
La Jolla, Calif., USA

Mechanisms and Implications of Capillary Endothelial Swelling and Luminal Narrowing in Low-Flow Ischemias

Key Words
Leukocyte
Hypertonic saline-dextran solution
Amiloride
No-reflow phenomenon
Microcirculation
Model analysis

Abstract
Decreased functional capillary density (FCD) is a characteristic of low-flow ischemia which often persists on reperfusion of a tissue even though supply blood flow is reestablished. Capillary narrowing is a possible mechanism for the reduced blood reflow through an increase of the hydraulic resistance of the capillary network. We attribute the narrowing to swollen endothelial cells, a condition that could be observed directly and was found to develop with blood acidosis in both hemorrhagic shock and intentional acid infusion. A computer model of blood flow in skeletal muscle was used to predict the impact of a 21% decrease in capillary luminal diameter on flow and leukocyte transit through the network. For hemorrhagic shock, reduction in blood flow due to capillary narrowing and lowered systemic pressure was offset by hemodilution causing a low-flow state. On reperfusion, flow could be restored if the narrowing was rectified by infusion of a hypertonic saline-dextran solution. Reinfusion with conventional Ringer's lactate only partially restored flow because of a persistent capillary narrowing. The rheological contribution of passive leukocytes added only a few percent to network resistance even with shock-narrowed capillaries. With leukocyte activation increased cell cytoplasmic viscosity caused prolonged transit times for leukocytes in the network with a concomitant elevation in resistance. We conclude that capillary narrowing is a mechanism of FCD reduction in reperfusion after low-flow ischemia, either by a direct effect on flow or by enhancing the transient plugging of leukocytes. Therapeutic strategies should aim to ameliorate or prevent capillary endothelial cell swelling, and to minimize the level of activated circulating leukocytes.

Introduction

Functional capillary density (FCD) is an index of blood flow giving the proportion of perfused nutrient capillaries in a specified tissue volume. FCD is relatively invariant over time in resting healthy tissues, but it can decrease dramatically in these same tissues under pathophysiological conditions. For example, following 4 h of complete ischemia and reperfusion in striated muscle, capillary perfusion was significantly impaired, the now well-documented 'no-reflow' phenomenon [1]. The mechanisms for the reduced FCD are not completely under-

Dr. Michelle C. Mazzoni
Institute for Biomedical Engineering, 0412
University of California, San Diego
La Jolla, CA 92093-0412 (USA)

0167-6865/95/0155-0265
$10.00/0

stood, but both hemodynamic and biochemical factors at the microcirculatory level probably play a role. One such local mechanism of potential importance is capillaries which become narrowed during the ischemic episode.

Only in the smallest blood vessels, i.e., the capillaries, is the thickness of the endothelial cell wall the same order of magnitude as the vessel diameter for flow. Swelling of the endothelium with encroachment into the vessel lumen has been shown for capillaries in skeletal muscle [2–4] and mesentery [5] during hemorrhagic shock (global low-flow ischemia). The acute decrease in luminal diameter would increase hydraulic flow resistance, thereby hindering reflow efforts. Moreover, narrowed capillaries may cause prolonged transient and long-term plugging of the leukocytes which are normally larger and much stiffer than the traversing red blood cells (RBCs).

It is the intent of this report to survey the findings made by the authors and coworkers over the past 5 years on endothelial cell swelling and capillary narrowing in low-flow ischemias and fluid reinfusion. The etiology and scope of this morphological alteration are discussed. Most recently, we have incorporated our in vivo measurements into a computer network model to predict the effects of individual mechanisms, specifically capillary narrowing, on microcirculatory blood flow [6]. The combined experimental and analytical approach provides a unique perspective into the impact of cellular events (e.g., endothelium edema) on whole organ function (e.g., FCD).

Materials and Methods

Animal Model

Experiments were carried out in the tenuissimus and gastrocnemius muscles of the rabbit hindlimb (male, New Zealand White, 0.8–1.6 kg) following 20% urethan anesthesia. Since the details of the animal and muscle preparations have been recently published [7], just a concise description of the methods will be given here with reference to the relevant study. The animals were implanted with up to four catheters depending on the objectives of the study. Carotid artery and jugular vein catheters were standard for blood removal (samples for analysis, hemorrhage) or microsphere injection and fluid infusion (saline, drugs, iso- and hypertonic solutions, hydrochloric acid). In addition, a catheter in the femoral artery allowed continuous monitoring of blood pressure or blood from it served as the reference organ in microsphere studies [6]. In some experiments, a femoral vein catheter was inserted to sample venous effluent from the hindlimb muscles. Supplementary doses of anesthesia (1–2 ml) were given as needed.

The tenuissimus muscle was surgically prepared as described by Lindbom et al. [8] and covered with a layer of sodium hyaluronate and Mylar film to eliminate gas and fluid exchange between tissue and the environment. The muscle and animal were maintained at 37 °C. Intravital microscopy with Köhler transillumination of the tenuissimus muscle allowed high-contrast observations of the microcirculation including single capillaries using high magnification (× 100, numeric aperture 1.20, depth of focus 0.36 μm). Both luminal and abluminal membranes of the endothelial wall could occasionally be visualized in capillaries which were on the top surface of the muscle and which deviated somewhat from the normal capillary arrangement of parallel alignment with the muscle fibers. Both conditions help to minimize light diffraction from surrounding structures and optimize resolution and contrast. Routinely, the capillary luminal diameter was measured as described below.

Microcirculatory blood flow was measured in the gastrocnemius muscle (in situ, underlying the tenuissimus muscle) using laser Doppler flowmetry (LDF) or a microsphere technique. The laser probe tip was positioned so that the signal represented, as near as possible, blood flow in the capillary network which can then be compared directly to the nutrient capillary flow as measured with microspheres. Such a comparison was made to investigate the degree of flow reduction in hemorrhagic shock.

Experimental Protocols

Low-flow ischemia was induced in the hindlimb muscles using two separate models. One was a standard hemorrhagic shock model in which the animal was acutely bled of 40% of its blood volume [2–4]. The procedure produced a protracted hypotension, metabolic acidosis, and global reduction in blood flow to nonessential organs such as skeletal muscle. The second model created a local reduction in blood flow to the hindlimb muscles by partial occlusion of the distal aorta with a balloon occluder [7]. The endpoint was a femoral arterial pressure of 15 mm Hg (normally about 70 mm Hg). Central hemodynamics were minimally affected by the occluder procedure.

To explore the possible mechanisms for capillary narrowing due to endothelial cell swelling, select pretreatments and/or treatments were performed. In one experimental study, the blood pH was reduced by intravenous infusion of hydrochloric acid (1.2 *M*, 4 ml/min/kg) to a level comparable to the metabolic acidosis of hemorrhagic shock [7]. For experiments in which endothelial cell swelling was found, further experiments had animals pretreated with the drug amiloride or one of its specific analogs which inhibit many transmembrane Na^+ transport systems. In particular, the amiloride analog 5-(N,N-hexamethylene)amiloride (HMA) which inhibits Na^+/H^+ exchange was given at a dose of 1 mg/kg 30 min prior to acid treatment [7] or hemorrhage [4].

The duration of the ischemic or acidotic episode was 1 h for all protocols. In the local low-flow ischemia experiments, spontaneous reperfusion was initiated after complete release of the occluder. In the hemorrhagic shock studies, the animals were reinfused with asanguinous fluids, either Ringer's lactate (RL) alone or in combination with an initial bolus of a hypertonic saline-dextran solution of 7.5% NaCl/6% dextran 70 (HSD) in a dose equal to one-seventh of the shed blood volume [3]. The reperfusion periods were followed for 30 min. The time course of this paradigm simulates the clinical trauma situation. Systemic parameters including arterial pressure, hematocrit, and blood gases were taken in the control period and at specified intervals in the ischemic, acidotic, and/or reperfusion periods.

Measurement of Capillary Diameter

Changes in luminal diameter were analyzed off-line from high-quality videotapes using a computer system that included customized software for random line length determination. The image had a

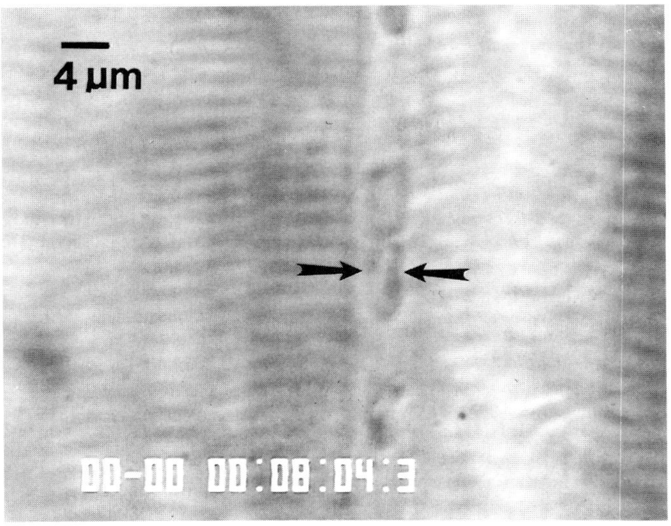

Fig. 1. Photograph of capillary in rabbit tenuissimus muscle. Luminal diameter was determined from the measurement of the widths of RBCs moving through the capillary in a single-file manner under moderate deformation.

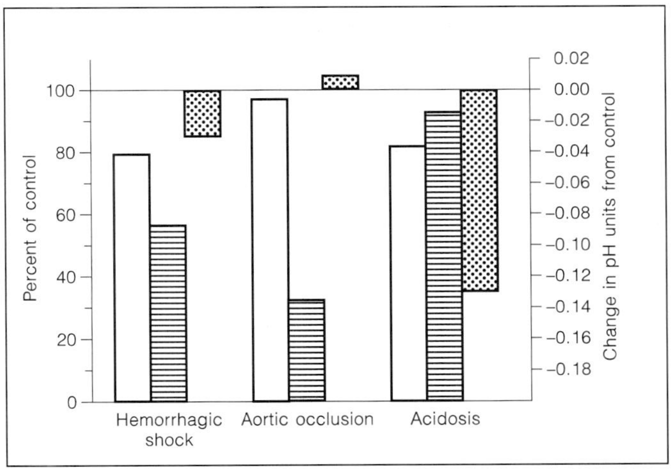

Fig. 2. Percent of control values for capillary luminal diameter (□) and LDF (▤) as compared to changes in arterial pH (▩) for three different experimental models: hemorrhagic shock (40% bleed), low-flow ischemia produced locally in the muscle by upstream aortic occlusion, and intentional blood acidosis. Capillary diameter correlates with arterial pH, but not with low flow per se.

calculated theoretical resolution of 0.3 µm and practical resolution of 0.4 µm [4], making it possible to discern the capillary wall; however, the contrast between the endothelial membranes and surrounding tissue varied unpredictably from sharp to hazy. So to quantify the distance between opposing luminal membranes, we measured the width of the dark contrasting RBCs which had momentarily slowed down or stopped in the capillary. Figure 1 shows that the RBCs (diameter of about 7 µm) must deform and adjust their shape just enough to fit through the smaller diameter capillaries (typically 4–5 µm) in skeletal muscle. We have documented that the RBCs are space-filling in the lumen [2] and by an independent means (fluorescently labeled plasma) that RBC width is an accurate indicator of luminal diameter both in control and hemorrhagic shock conditions [4]. In sections of capillaries when both opposing luminal and abluminal membranes could be viewed, the thickness of the endothelium was assessed. Optimal resolution of the endothelial wall was achieved on a focal plane of view slightly above that for the RBCs in the capillary lumen because the × 100 objective has a shallow depth of focus (0.36 µm) [4].

Computer Model for Capillary Network Blood Flow

The effects of capillary luminal narrowing, as well as changes in other hemodynamic factors in ischemia/reperfusion (I/R) (e.g., blood pressure, hematocrit), on microcirculatory blood flow were examined using a computer model [6]. The model is based on a typical microvascular unit in skeletal muscle with the capillary network fed by a single arteriole and drained by a single venule. Model blood flow is a function of the pressure gradient across the network, the dimensions of the vessels in the network, the blood viscosity in each vessel, the network leukocrit, and the leukocyte cytoplasmic viscosity. The amount that these parameters changed during hemorrhagic shock and reperfusion was provided by the in vivo data reviewed here and previously reported [2, 3, 6]. Of interest is the incorporation of leukocyte rheology into the model. The greater cytoplasmic viscosity of the leukocytes imposes an added network resistance compared to the resistance imposed by RBCs alone. First, there is a momentary plugging of the leukocyte at the capillary entrance which precludes flow into that vessel for a span of time inversely proportional to the pressure gradient across the cell. Then, once inside the capillary lumen, the presence of each leukocyte contributes a higher resistance in the segment of vessel it occupies. Leukocyte adhesion is assumed not to occur in the capillaries (no evidence has shown otherwise), so theoretically at least, leukocyte plugs will not be permanent unless there are conditions of zero blood flow.

Results

Capillary Narrowing – Endothelial Cell Swelling

Luminal diameters of capillaries in the tenuissimus muscle were observed under the conditions of hemorrhagic shock, local low-flow ischemia in the muscle, and systemic blood acidosis. We originally reported in 1989 the in vivo finding of capillary narrowing in hemorrhagic shock owing to swollen endothelial cells [2]. Evidence for the occurrence of edematous endothelium has since been strengthened with high-contrast direct visualization [4]. Because hemorrhagic shock induces alterations in both flow and blood pH in the muscle, we devised separate models to study each factor as a potential mechanism for narrowing. Figure 2 shows changes in capillary luminal diameter, muscle blood flow as measured by LDF, and arterial pH after 1 h of either acidosis or low-flow ischemia by aortic occlusion, compared to the original shock data. A narrowing of diameter to 82% of the control value occurred with intentional blood acidosis (comparable to 79% of the control value in shock), but there was no significant diameter change with just flow reduction [7]. In the acidosis capillaries, a thickening of the endothelium was apparent on visual examination at the appropriate focal plane of a couple of capillaries with a clearly defined abluminal membrane. Spontaneous reperfusion of the muscle (with systemic blood of normal pH) after release of the aortic occluder produced no detectable narrowing in the ischemic capillaries [7].

Interventions of Endothelium Volume Increase

Pretreatment with the amiloride analog HMA to block Na^+/H^+ exchange completely prevented capillary narrowing in those cases in which it was found to occur, i.e., hemorrhagic shock [4] and systemic blood acidosis [7]. Once the endothelium was swollen, however, HMA or intravenous sodium bicarbonate (to correct arterial pH) had no effect on restoring volume [unpubl. data]. Since pretreatment is often not a feasible clinical approach, ways to minimize or reverse cell swelling were addressed upon flow restitution. It was found that fluid reinfusion with HSD completely rectified capillary hemodynamics including vessel diameter, whereas the conventional isotonic RL only modestly improved flow and was ineffective in restoring capillary diameter [3].

Implications of Capillary Narrowing

With the use of a computer model, changes in network blood flow were determined under conditions of hemorrhagic shock and fluid reinfusion. Specifically, capillary luminal narrowing of 21% was found to reduce flow by 13 to 36% with other factors unchanged, depending on whether one-half or all the capillaries in the proximal section of the network were assigned decreased diameters [6]. For the case of shock, a narrowing of one-half of the proximal capillaries combined with the lowered systemic pressure gave a very low flow which was offset in part by a relative flow increase due to hemodilution (decreased viscosity). The model prediction of a 50% flow reduction in shock (half of proximal capillaries narrowed) was validated by both microsphere and LDF results [6]. On reperfusion, the model agreed with the experimental LDF findings of partial flow recovery with RL (persistent capillary luminal narrowing) and full flow recovery with HSD (complete rectification of capillary luminal diameters) [6]. The model analysis further predicted that leukocytes contribute minimally to total network resistance, even in the low-flow shock state, unless the cells are activated with an attendant increased cytoplasmic viscosity [6].

Discussion

Numerous studies on I/R injury appear in the literature because the problem pertains to many prevalent cardiovascular diseases, vascular and tissue transplant surgeries, and trauma situations. In particular, the role of leukocytes in no-reflow (FCD reduction) after I/R has been a heavily pursued research topic. Much less attention has been given to acute decreases in capillary diameter as a cause of flow impairment, except in a capacity to impede leukocyte circulation. Although the impact of leukocyte plugging and activation on microcirculatory blood flow is not the primary focus of this report, perusal of such studies indirectly lends support to the concept of capillary luminal narrowing as a potentially important and distinct mechanism of the no-reflow phenomenon.

Leukocytes can conceivably bring about tissue damage by limiting nutrient blood flow or by releasing cytotoxic mediators (e.g., proteolytic enzymes, oxygen free radicals) into the tissue after endothelial cell-mediated activation and emigration (the so-called inflammatory response). Activation of the circulating leukocytes exacerbates the situation because activated leukocytes are stiffer and thus more likely to become trapped in capillaries, and the premature liberation of toxins can degenerate the delicate endothelial cells. In I/R studies in the brain, the recovery of blood flow after an ischemic insult was only slightly improved when the leukocytes were removed from the blood prior to the ischemia [9, 10]. But in an isolated skeletal muscle model of I/R, the presence of leukocytes was associated with a twofold increase in vascular resistance as compared to leukocyte-depleted blood [11]. This result suggests a direct hemodynamic effect of the leukocytes via transient plugging and slower transit times in the capillaries, but whether cellular activation contributed to this effect is not known since the extent of leukocyte activation was not measured. Our model computations find the additional network resistance due to inactivated leukocytes at physiological concentration to be less than 2%.

Different approaches have been tried to elucidate the involvement of activated neutrophils in I/R injury. Animals pretreated with the monoclonal antibody to CD18, the leukocyte receptor molecule responsible for firm adhesion, were found to have mitigated cellular organ injury and 100% survival on reperfusion with shed blood compared to gross cellular damage and 27% survival in untreated animals [12]. So it appears that just the physical presence of the leukocytes is not an exclusive factor in promoting I/R injury – leukocyte activation must also occur. Our model computations concur with this view from a hemodynamic standpoint, in that leukocytes do add significantly to organ resistance only if they are activated and hence stiffer. Further, Menger et al. [1], using a 4-hour tourniquet ischemia model in skeletal muscle, showed that if oxygen-derived free radical formation was prevented (with allopurinol) or if these toxic substances were scavenged (with superoxide dismutase), the percentage of nonperfused capillaries relative to control after 24 h decreased (40% vs. 65% in untreated group). Even though the FCD was improved with treatment, there were still many capillaries with no-reflow which had initially been perfused. Therefore, on the basis of these cited leukocyte results, mechanisms other than leukocyte rheology and biochemical activity must also be operative in the development of I/R injury.

To recapitulate, leukocytes alone cannot explain the no-reflow phenomenon. Capillary luminal narrowing is a real event capable of producing large network flow decreases through the strong dependence of flow on the inverse fourth power of vessel diameter. The narrowing we found in skeletal muscle capillaries during hemorrhagic shock and systemic blood acidosis was attributed to a swelling of the endothelium which comprises the capillary wall. Only a small number of the observed capillaries had the specific optical features needed to facilitate discernment of the swollen walls. In these examples, the outer abluminal diameter did not change dimension with just the inner luminal diameter becoming smaller as the wall thickness increased [4]. Since we have usually only inferred swelling from the measurement of luminal diameter, it has been a point of contention when stated unequivocally that endothelial cells swell in hemorrhagic shock and acidosis, despite some select examples. For the purpose of exploring mechanisms for no-reflow, however, it suffices to state that capillary narrowing itself is a mechanism for microcirculatory flow impairment.

Capillary narrowing could be caused by edematous endothelial cells, as we propose, or vessel compression. Compliant capillaries could narrow in response to a lowered intraluminal pressure or an increased tissue pressure. The time history of these pressures was not determined in our models, so a direct relation to capillary diameter changes is not possible. In hemorrhagic shock, the narrowing which developed over an hour was not apparent at 10–15 min into shock [unpubl. data], despite an expected drop in capillary pressure [13]. Moreover, animal pretreatment with the amiloride analog HMA prevented the narrowing in shock [4], and in a model where blood flow was lowered by an upstream pressure reduction, there was again no narrowing [7]. These results taken together along with the measurement of a fixed outer capillary diameter [4] discount elastic behavior as the explanation for the narrowing we observe. Specifically, we have found that it is the acidotic nature of the blood, and not the reduction in blood flow per se, which is responsible for cell swelling in the models of low-flow ischemia we investigated (fig. 2) [7].

Swollen capillary endothelium has been demonstrated in skeletal muscle after complete ischemia [14] and in mesentery after a combined trauma and hemorrhagic shock insult [5]. This latter study just published concluded that endothelial cells swell in capillaries with an open lumen (mean endothelial height increase of about 70%), but not in capillaries with the lumen blocked by blood cells (no perfusion). It seems unlikely, as the authors speculate, that rigid RBCs keep the lumen open. Possibly in those capillaries without flow, the endothelium was not exposed to the circulating systemic blood acidosis which would be expected in this shock model (blood pH was not measured). Support for endothelial cell swelling with blood acidosis comes from in vitro studies which show cell swelling with extracellular acidosis [15, 16]. Furthermore, we found the same degree of capillary narrowing (i.e., endothelial cell swelling) when we induced blood acidosis as compared to hemorrhagic shock [7]. The narrowing was entirely prevented by pretreatment with the amiloride analog HMA [7], which prevents cells from regulating intracellular pH [17].

Capillary narrowing clearly diminishes network blood flow, and it may also disturb the distribution of flow to the point that some capillaries cease to have flow. This decrease in the FCD of a tissue, which describes the no-reflow phenomenon observed after I/R, could occur if there exists a large disparity in hydraulic resistances among capillaries branching from the same arterial tree or parent capillary. RBCs and leukocytes will take the path of least resistance, thereby creating preferential flow pathways in the microcirculation. Leukocytes, especially if activated, will have much longer transit times and may plug in capillaries with now reduced luminal diameters even if only a small section of the capillary is affected, i.e., the swelling of endothelial cells is sporadic or pronounced in the nuclear region of the cell. Thus, capillary narrowing could reduce FCD directly or indirectly by enhancing the entrapment of leukocytes.

In the clinical scenario, prevention of endothelium swelling through pretreatment with drugs like amiloride and its analogs may be practical if imminent ischemia is anticipated, e.g., surgery requiring the clamping of blood vessels. This is the exception for most situations of I/R, however, so swelling must be addressed after the fact. To date, the only effective treatment is the use of HSD as an osmotic maneuver to pull water from edematous endothelial cells [18]. After 1 h of hemorrhagic shock, HSD completely restored capillary luminal diameters whereas conventional RL had no effect [3]. Model calculations agree with experimental LDF results that HSD also quickly reestablished microcirculatory blood flow, with RL producing only a sluggish and partial flow recovery [6]. Nolte et al. [19] showed that HSD administered before reperfusion of ischemic striated muscle reopened narrowed capillaries and preserved FCD. Also and interestingly, leukocyte-endothelium adhesive interaction was attenuated, presumably due to an inhibitory effect exerted by the dextran. Such down-regulation could be beneficial in mitigating I/R injury associated with activated leukocytes.

In conclusion, a combined experimental and analytical approach has been presented to substantiate the importance of capillary luminal narrowing as an individual mechanism for FCD reduction. Capillary narrowing could contribute to the deleterious hemodynamic and biochemical effects of activated leukocytes. The underlying endothelial cell swelling which develops as a consequence of systemic blood acidosis can be prevented by pretreatment with HMA to block cellular pH regulation or reversed with HSD. As a final point, to circumvent the development of no-reflow and its related secondary clinical complications, consideration should be made to maintain microcirculatory flow levels with blood at normal pH.

References

1 Menger MD, Steiner D, Messmer K: Microvascular ischemia-reperfusion injury in striated muscle: Significance of 'no-reflow'. Am J Physiol 1992;263:H1892–H1900.
2 Mazzoni MC, Borgström P, Intaglietta M, Arfors KE: Luminal narrowing and endothelial cell swelling in skeletal muscle capillaries during hemorrhagic shock. Circ Shock 1989;29:27–39.
3 Mazzoni MC, Borgström P, Intaglietta M, Arfors KE: Capillary narrowing in hemorrhagic shock is rectified by hyperosmotic saline-dextran reinfusion. Circ Shock 1990;31:407–418.
4 Mazzoni MC, Intaglietta M, Cragoe EJ, Arfors KE: Amiloride-sensitive Na^+ pathways in capillary endothelial cell swelling during hemorrhagic shock. J Appl Physiol 1992;73:1467–1473.
5 Kretschmar K, Engelhardt T: Swelling of capillary endothelial cells contributes to traumatic hemorrhagic shock-induced microvascular injury: A morphologic and morphometric analysis. Int J Microcirc Clin Exp 1994;14:45–49.
6 Mazzoni MC, Warnke KC, Arfors KE, Skalak TC: Capillary hemodynamics in hemorrhagic shock and reperfusion: In vivo and model analysis. Am J Physiol 1994;267:H1928–H1935.
7 Mazzoni MC, Cragoe EJ, Arfors KE: Systemic blood acidosis in low-flow ischemia induces capillary luminal narrowing. Int J Microcirc 1994;14:144–150.
8 Lindbom L, Tuma RF, Arfors KE: Influence of oxygen on perfused capillary density and capillary red cell velocity in rabbit skeletal muscle. Microvasc Res 1980;19:197–208.
9 Bednar MM, Raymond S, McAuliffe T, Lodge PA, Gross CE: The role of neutrophils and platelets in a rabbit model of thromboembolic stroke. Stroke 1991;22:44–50.
10 Grøgaard B, Schürer L, Gerdin B, Arfors KE: Delayed hypoperfusion after incomplete forebrain ischemia in the rat: The role of polymorphonuclear leukocytes. J Cereb Blood Flow Metab 1989;9:500–505.
11 Korthuis RJ, Grisham MB, Granger DN: Leukocyte depletion attenuates vascular injury in postischemic skeletal muscle. Am J Physiol 1988;254:H823–H827.
12 Vedder NB, Winn RK, Rice CL, Chi EY, Arfors KE, Harlan JM: A monoclonal antibody to the adherence-promoting leukocyte glycoprotein, CD18, reduces organ injury and improves survival from hemorrhagic shock and resuscitation in rabbits. J Clin Invest 1988;81:939–944.
13 Zweifach BW: Mechanisms of blood flow and fluid exchange in microvessels: Hemorrhagic hypotension model. Anesthesiology 1974;41:157–168.
14 Gidlöf A, Lewis DH, Hammersen F: The effect of prolonged total ischemia on the ultrastructure of human skeletal muscle capillaries: A morphometric analysis. Int J Microcirc Clin Exp 1987;7:67–86.
15 Jakubovicz DE, Klip A: Lactic acid-induced swelling in C6 glial cells via Na^+/H^+ exchange. Brain Res 1989;485:215–224.
16 Kempski O, Staub F, Jansen M, Schödel F, Baethmann A: Glial swelling during extracellular acidosis in vitro. Stroke 1988;19:385–392.
17 Cala PM, Anderson SE, Cragoe EJ: Na/H exchange-dependent cell volume and pH regulation and disturbances. Comp Biochem Physiol A 1988;90:551–555.
18 Mazzoni MC, Borgström P, Arfors KE, Intaglietta M: Dynamic fluid redistribution in hyperosmotic resuscitation of hypovolemic hemorrhage. Am J Physiol 1988;255:H629–H637.
19 Nolte D, Bayer M, Lehr HA, Becker M, Krombach F, Kreimeier U, Messmer K: Attenuation of postischemic microvascular disturbances in striated muscle by hyperosmolar saline dextran. Am J Physiol 1992;263:H1411–H1416.

Int J Microcirc 1995;15:271–275

D.W. Slaaf[a]
J. Bosman[a]
G.J. Tangelder[b]
M.G.A. oude Egbrink[b]
R.S. Reneman[b]

Departments of
[a] Biophysics and
[b] Physiology, Cardiovascular Research Institute Maastricht, University of Limburg, Maastricht, The Netherlands

Oxygen- and Pressure-Dependent Functional Capillary Density in Rabbit Tenuissimus Muscle

Key Words
Intravital microscopy
Capillary diameter
Aorta occlusion
Capillary density
Oxygen

Abstract
Perfusion of capillaries was investigated in the tenuissimus muscle of young anesthetized New Zealand White rabbits during control conditions, complete aorta occlusion, and reactive hyperemia at various local oxygen tensions. Capillaries were visualized with bright-field microscopy. The number of capillaries perfused under experimental conditions was compared with that during control conditions. Capillary diameter was measured to assess whether the interventions caused changes in luminal diameter. During control conditions at a local pO_2 of about 20 mm Hg, capillary perfusion fluctuates; instantaneous capillary density is smaller than anatomical capillary density. When the aorta is (partially) occluded, capillary perfusion becomes continuous and instantaneous capillary density equals anatomical capillary density. The latter is also observed during the early phase of reactive hyperemia, prior to the reappearance of flowmotion. Capillary diameter is not invariant during these interventions, but decreases by 8% during occlusion and increases by 12% during reactive hyperemia. The concomitant change in perimeter and cross-sectional area should be factored in with functional capillary density, when tissue exchange surface area or volume flow are considered. When during control conditions, the muscle becomes locally (under the microscope lens) exposed to a higher oxygen tension, capillary diameter does not change. However, the relative number of capillaries perfused at complete aorta occlusion is unity at low local oxygen, and diminishes with increasing local oxygen to become 0 at an oxygen tension of about 70 mm Hg. In preparations in which capillary diameter is not invariant under the experimental conditions, functional capillary density can only be used to compare the number of perfused capillaries with the number of capillaries anatomically present. Capillary diameter has to be factored in when tissue perfusion or exchange surface area are considered.

Dick W. Slaaf, PhD
Department of Biophysics
Cardiovascular Research Institute Maastricht
University of Limburg, PO Box 616
6200 MD Maastricht (The Netherlands)

0167–6865/95/0155–0271
$10.00/0

Introduction

Capillary perfusion is an important determinant of tissue oxygenation [1]. The number (and length) of capillaries in a tissue are a measure for perfusion and exchange capacity. Anatomical capillary density is usually defined as the number of capillaries in a unit of cross-sectional area or volume of tissue [2]. The anatomical presence of capillaries does not necessarily imply that these capillaries actually carry flow and are involved in the perfusion or exchange process. A certain number of capillaries may be deprived of blood flow. This spatial heterogeneity in perfusion may vary with time. An important effector of this temporal heterogeneity of capillary perfusion is vasomotion, i.e., the more or less rhythmic diameter variation in (terminal) arterioles [3–5]. Counting only the capillaries attended by red blood cells (RBCs) in stained cross sections and comparing that with the total number of capillaries present is not a suitable method to assess the fraction of actually perfused capillaries, because capillaries containing RBCs may not be perfused, and variations in hematocrit due to vasomotion in the terminal arterioles may result in perfused capillaries without RBCs. Therefore, functional capillary density is often used to describe the number of capillaries in a certain volume of tissue that are being perfused with RBCs [6]. One should bear in mind, however, that according to this definition, transport and exchange capacity can change without a change in functional capillary density, for example, when capillary diameters are not invariant. This is not necessarily the case. Davis [7], and Bouskela and Wiederhielm [8] demonstrated that in connective tissue in the bat wing, capillaries are distensible and that they actually change diameter at variations in transmural pressure within the physiological range. This implies that functional capillary density is not the only variable determining tissue flow capacity or exchange surface area.

Data obtained from preliminary experiments suggest that in skeletal muscle also, capillary diameter might vary not only with transmural pressure, but also with local oxygen tension; capillary perfusion appeared to be strongly related to locally applied oxygen tension, while the arterioles were always open to perfusion [9].

In this paper, studies are described in which perfusion and diameter of capillaries of the tenuissimus muscle of young anesthetized rabbits were investigated during control, low perfusion pressure, and subsequent reactive hyperemia. Special attention was paid to possible changes in diameter and the influence of oxygen on the relative number of capillaries still perfused during complete aorta occlusion. The findings are discussed in relation to perfusion and exchange capacity.

Materials and Methods

Experiments were performed on young (5–6 weeks, 0.8–1.1 kg weight) New Zealand White rabbits of both sexes. All experimental procedures were approved by the Institutional Animal Care and Use Committee of the University of Limburg. The rabbits were premedicated with diazepam (5 mg; Valium, Roche), intramuscularly. Half an hour later, anesthesia was induced by injection of urethane (4 ml of a 20% solution) through a lateral ear vein. Anesthesia was maintained throughout the experiment with additional doses of urethane (about 0.4 ml/30 min) through a catheter in the right femoral vein, if necessary.

A trachea cannula was inserted to facilitate breathing. Arterial blood pressure (external pressure transducer, model CP-01, CTC) and heart rate were recorded through a catheter placed in the right carotid artery.

Perfusion pressure in the tenuissimus muscle was reduced by inflating a cuff placed around the aorta distal to the renal arteries. When the cuff was inflated, the aorta occluded completely. Arterial pressure downstream of the cuff was measured through a catheter in the femoral artery of the (contralateral) right hindlimb. Both arterial catheters were perfused with saline (0.9% NaCl) at a rate of 2.5 ml/h to keep them patent.

In the control situation, mean carotid artery pressure was between 70 and 107 mm Hg, and mean femoral artery pressure was between 67 and 105 mm Hg. Heart rate varied between 252 and 380 beats/min. Body temperature was kept at 38 °C throughout the experiment. Arterial blood gas and pH values were assessed with an acid-base analyzer (model ABL 3, Radiometer, Copenhagen, Denmark). Arterial pO_2 and PCO_2 were 74 (58–88) and 38 (34–45) mm Hg, respectively, and pH was 7.37 (7.28–7.45).

Tenuissimus Muscle

The preparation procedure has been described in detail elsewhere [10]. In short, the muscle of the left hindpaw was carefully exposed for in situ microscopic observation. The muscle itself was not touched, and fascia, tendons, innervation, and supplying and draining blood vessels were left intact. During the preparation, the muscle was superfused with a 0.9% NaCl solution at room temperature (20–23 °C). Subsequently, the leg was positioned in a sealable box to enable control of the gas environment. A light pipe was placed underneath the muscle for transillumination [10].

The box was sealed and a gas mixture of 95% N_2 and 5% CO_2 was led through the box. Muscle superfusion in the box was performed at 37 °C with a Krebs solution (composition in m*M*: $NaHCO_3$, 25; KH_2PO_4, 1.2; KCl, 4.8; $CaCl_2$, 2.5; $MgSO_4$, 1.2; NaCl, 118.4). pH was kept at 7.4 ± 0.5, by bubbling with a gas mixture containing 5% CO_2. The remainder of this gas composition could be varied between 95% N_2 and 95% O_2, keeping pH constant. The muscle was allowed to recover and equilibrate to each specific experimental condition for a period of about 30 min. Applying a superfusion solution with a certain oxygen tension to the muscle, while passing a gas mixture without oxygen through the box led to a local oxygen concentration in the solution under the microscope objective of 89% compared to the concentration in the superfusion solution just prior to entrance into the box. The remainder of the muscle was exposed to low (<20 mm Hg) oxygen tension due to oxygen washout from the superfusate by the oxygen-free gas mixture flowing through the box. The oxygen concentrations reported in the results section are the corrected ones. Oxygen is known to induce vasoconstriction in arterioles leading to cessation of capillary perfusion [11]. In the present experiments with the local application of oxygen, however, capillary flow was usually present. This suggests that the terminal arterioles were located outside the area effectively exposed to the higher oxygen tensions.

Microscope and Experimental Procedure

A Leitz microscope adapted for telescopic imaging was used for microscopic observations [12]. Images were projected on a TV camera, displayed on a video monitor, and stored on videotape. Final optical magnification at the front plane of the camera was × 52 or × 104, using salt water immersion objectives of × 25 (numerical aperture 0.6) and × 50 (numerical aperture 1.0), respectively. This yielded a field of view on the monitor of 230 and 115 μm horizontal width, respectively. Transillumination was performed with a 100-watt mercury arc with appropriate heat filters, a fiber optic, and a condensor system positioned in front of the light pipe [10]. Neutral density filters were used to adjust light levels to the lowest level still yielding good images.

Video recordings were made before, during, and after complete aorta occlusion at various local oxygen tensions. After a control period of at least 2 min, the aorta was completely occluded for 2 min. Within about 20 s, occlusion resulted in a low femoral artery pressure (4–22 mm Hg). This variability in femoral artery pressures attained is due to collateral circulation. The time interval between successive occlusions was at least 5 min.

Two sets of experiments were performed. In the first set, we assessed the relative number of capillaries per field of view that were still perfused with RBCs during complete aorta occlusion, compared to the control, using the × 25 objective. Each field studied contained 3–6 capillaries. At control arterial pressure, flow was present in all capillaries. The experiments were performed at various local oxygen tensions. Counts of capillaries carrying flow were performed off-line.

In another set of experiments, we measured capillary diameter along short segments of a capillary. We selected capillaries that (1) ran for their longest part parallel to the muscle fibers, (2) contained RBCs flowing in single file, and (3) were in focus for a considerable length. The capillaries were oriented vertically on the monitor screen using a K-mirror. Using the × 50 objective lens, recordings of capillaries were made during control (2 min), occlusion (2 min), and reactive hyperemia after release of the occluder (2 min) at various local oxygen tensions. Resolution of the microscope-camera-monitor system was about 0.3 μm.

Diameter Measurements

Inner capillary diameter was assessed off-line using a home-built image-shearing device [13]. Measurements were performed at several sites (4–6, clearly in focus) along each capillary and repeated at various moments during a control period (4–6 times), aorta occlusion (4–6 times), and reactive hyperemia (4–8 times). During the control period, we calculated the mean control diameter for a given segment as the mean of the various sites at the various moments. To estimate the consequences for resistance to flow, we calculated equivalent diameter as the mean of the instantaneous equivalent-diameter values. Equivalent diameter is defined as the diameter of a uniform vessel having the same resistance to flow as the vessel studied. It can be calculated from the following relationship [14]:

$$D_{eq} = \left[\frac{n}{\sum_{i=1}^{n} D_i^{-4}} \right]^{1/4}$$

where D_i is capillary diameter at site i, and n the number of observations along the segment. Equivalent diameter is a measure of the influence of the geometry on vascular resistance.

Relative D_{eq} (compared to control) was used to calculate the (relative) resistance, which is proportional to (relative) D_{eq}^{-4}.

Blood Cell Velocity Measurements

Blood cell velocities in the capillaries were measured off-line, using the dual-window technique [15] and the Capiflow temporal-correlation software. Settings of the windows and the correlation process were optimized for each measurement.

Data Presentation and Statistical Analysis

Data are presented as medians and ranges. For statistical analysis, we used the SPSS-PC+ statistical package (SPSS Inc., Chicago, Ill., USA). The Mann-Whitney U test was used to compare independent data groups. Paired data were compared using the Wilcoxon signed-rank test. In all tests the level of significance was set at 5%.

Results and Discussion

In young rabbit tenuissimus muscle, capillaries exhibit flow motion [16], i.e., more or less rhythmic changes in capillary blood cell velocity (fig. 1). We observed a fast- (median cycle length 4.6 s; 2.7–6.9 s) and a slow-wave (24 s; 9–38 s) component. Oude Vrielink et al. [17] found that the number of perfused capillaries originating from a certain terminal arteriole during control did not differ from the number during complete vasodilation during superfusion with aenosine (10^{-4} *M*). They also demonstrated that all terminal arterioles were perfused, albeit intermittently. These data indicate that no anatomical recruitment is present in the tenuissimus muscle of young rabbits. When considered over a prolonged period of time, functional capillary density is in this case 100% of anatomical capillary density. Instantaneous functional capillary density, however, never equals anatomical capillary density due to the presence of flowmotion. For total flow calculations through a tissue, one takes this into account by multiplying functional capillary density by mean velocity.

Reduction of perfusion pressure initially leads to increased vasomotion and flowmotion amplitude [5], and subsequently to disappearance of vasomotion and to continuous perfusion of the capillaries (this study). When the

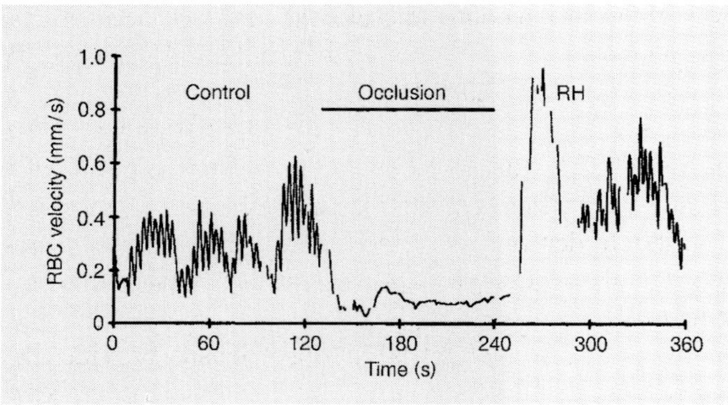

1

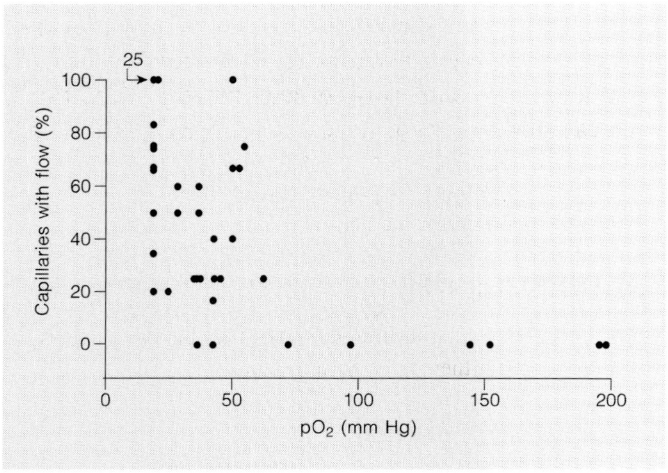

2

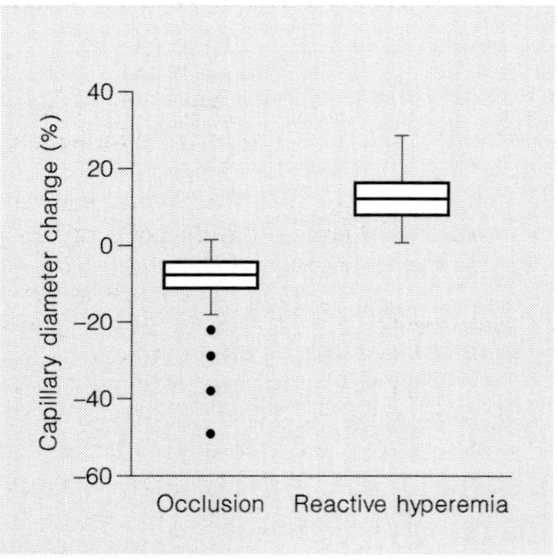

3

Fig. 1. Tracing of RBC velocity in a capillary during control, occlusion, and subsequent reactive hyperemia (RH). Note the fast and slow wave components of the flowmotion. During the early peak of RH, assessment of velocity is an approximation.

Fig. 2. The relative number of capillaries per field of view carrying flow (as compared with control situation = 100%) as a function of local oxygen tension. The number 25 at the top left indicates 25 data points at that position.

Fig. 3. Changes in capillary diameter (relative to control diameter) during occlusion and reactive hyperemia. Box plots represent median, interquartile range, and total range. The dots indicate stray values.

muscle is exposed to low oxygen in the superfusion solution, flow remains present in almost all capillaries during low perfusion pressure (fig. 2). At any moment during this intervention, instantaneous functional capillary density now approximates anatomical capillary density. To keep perfusion at the required level at these low driving pressures, all capillaries have been made available for continuous perfusion in order to obtain the lowest resistance: temporal recruitment.

During reactive hyperemia following release of the occluder, capillary flow velocity becomes very high and subsequently returns to control values. During the later phase of reactive hyperemia, flowmotion reappears (fig. 1). Therefore, instantaneous capillary density during reactive hyperemia equals anatomical capillary density until flowmotion reappears.

Functional capillary density is usually used as an indicator to compare flow-carrying capacity or exchange surface area in various situations. In the case of invariant capillary diameter, multiplication of functional capillary density with mean capillary flow velocity suffices to estimate total tissue flow, while capillary density can be used directly to compare exchange surface area. If, however, there are differences in capillary diameter between the situations under investigation (fig. 3), one should take these differences into account. During occlusion, mean equivalent capillary diameter is reduced by 8%, leading to a reduction in exchange surface area of 8% and in flow-carrying capacity of 16%. During reactive hyperemia, mean equivalent diameter is increased by 12% as compared with the control. In this situation, the increase in exchange surface area is 12% and that in flow-carrying capacity, 24%. Therefore, a mere comparison of capillary densities leads to considerable errors.

When the muscle is exposed to higher *local* oxygen tensions under the microscope lens only, capillary diameter during complete aorta occlusion decreased to the same extent as it did without local exposure to high oxygen tension. Therefore, local exposure to higher oxygen tensions does not influence capillary diameter and cross-sectional area. Under these same conditions, the number of capillaries still carrying flow (during complete aorta occlusion) decreased with increasing oxygen tension. When locally exposed to high oxygen tension (more than 70 mm Hg), occlusion of the aorta led to cessation of flow in virtually all capillaries. Instantaneous functional capillary density was reduced to 0% of anatomical capillary density. At intermediate local oxygen tensions, a graded reduction in (instantaneous) functional capillary density was present (fig. 2). The presence of local oxygen causes instantaneous functional capillary density to deviate from anatomical capillary density. Local application of oxygen only influences instantaneous functional capillary density, but not capillary diameter.

It is known that functional capillary density is oxygen dependent. When a muscle is completely exposed to high oxygen levels, the arterioles gradually constrict, which results in a gradually increasing number of downstream capillaries where flow ceases [11]. Sullivan and Johnson [18] demonstrated that when a rat skeletal muscle is completely exposed to 66 mm Hg of oxygen tension, arterioles constrict slightly (5–10%) at control pressures. When arterial pressure was reduced to 40 mm Hg at the same oxygen tension, no changes in arteriolar diameter occurred: the autoregulatory dilation was abolished in all arterioles. In our experiments, however, we demonstrated that when exposed to increasing (up to 50 mm Hg) levels of locally applied oxygen tension, the arterioles are all open and effectively dilated by 12% (1–43%) at complete aorta occlusion, probably because they are located outside the effective oxygenation zone.

In the evaluation of experiments on tissue perfusion in which capillary diameter is not invariant, one should not only take into account anatomical capillary density and the relative number of perfused capillaries, but also the relative capillary diameter. Functional capillary density should only be used to compare the number of capillaries perfused with the number of capillaries anatomically present. For tissue flow and tissue exchange surface area, one should demonstrate the invariance of capillary diameter if only functional capillary density is used for comparison.

In conclusion, functional capillary density provides the number of capillaries accessible to flow with respect to the process under study. Besides the relative number of capillaries perfused, one should also assess capillary diameter (and where appropriate capillary perimeter or cross-sectional area) for comparison of experimental conditions, since capillaries are not necessarily invariant in diameter.

Acknowledgments

The authors are indebted to Miss Sabrina van Velzen and Mr. Rinus Alewijnse for their technical assistance.

References

1 Renkin EM: Control of microcirculation and blood-tissue exchange; in Renkin EM, Michel CC (eds): Handbook of Physiology, section 2: The Cardiovascular System. Bethesda, American Physiological Society, 1984, vol 4: Microcirculation, part 2, pp 627–687.

2 Hudlicka O: Development of microcirculation: Capillary growth and adaptation; in Renkin EM, Michel CC (eds): Handbook of Physiology, section 2: The Cardiovascular System. Bethesda, American Physiological Society, 1984, vol 4: Microcirculation, part 1, pp 165–216.

3 Slaaf DW, Tangelder GJ, Teirlinck HC, Reneman RS: Arteriolar vasomotion and pressure reduction in rabbit tenuissimus muscle. Microvasc Res 1987;33:71–80.

4 Meyer JU, Lindbom L, Intaglietta M: Coordinated diameter oscillations at arteriolar bifurcations in skeletal muscle. Am J Physiol 1987; 253:H568–H573.

5 Oude Vrielink HHE, Slaaf DW, Tangelder GJ, Reneman RS: Changes in vasomotion pattern and local arteriolar resistance during stepwise pressure reduction. Eur J Physiol 1989;414: 571–578.

6 Damon DH, Duling BR: Distribution of capillary blood flow in the microcirculation of the hamster: An in vivo study using epifluorescent microscopy. Microvasc Res 1984;27:81–95.

7 Davis MJ: Microvascular control of capillary pressure during increases in local arterial and venous pressure. Am J Physiol 1988;254: H772–H784.

8 Bouskela E, Wiederhielm CA: Distensibility of capillaries in the bat wing. Blood Vessels 1989; 26:325–334.

9 Bosman J, Slaaf DW, Tangelder GJ, Reneman RS: Oxygen tension influences the flow cessation phenomenon and capillary diameter in skeletal muscle capillaries of anesthetized rabbits (abstract). Int J Microcirc Clin Exp 1992; 11(suppl 1):42.

10 Reneman RS, Slaaf DW, Lindbom L, Tangelder GJ, Arfors KE: Muscle blood flow disturbances produced by simultaneously elevated venous and total muscle tissue pressure. Microvasc Res 1980;20:307–318.

11 Lindbom L, Tuma RF, Arfors KE: Influence of oxygen on perfused capillary density and capillary red cell velocity in rabbit skeletal muscle. Microvasc Res 1980;19:197–208.

12 Slaaf DW, Alewijnse R, Wayland H: Use of telescopic imaging in intravital microscopy: A simple solution for conventional microscopes. Int J Microcirc Clin Exp 1982;1:121–134.

13 Intaglietta M, Tompkins WR: Microvascular measurements by video image shearing and splitting. Microvasc Res 1973;5:309–312.

14 Miles FP, Nuttall AL: Microvessel diameter estimation: Error bias correction of serial measurements. Biorheology 1991;28:315–332.

15 Slaaf DW, Arts T, Jeurens TJM, Tangelder GJ, Reneman RS: Electronic measurement of red blood cell velocity and volume flow in microvessels; in Chayen J, Bitensky L (eds): Investigative Microtechniques in Medicine and Biology. New York, Dekker, 1984, pp 327–364.

16 Tangelder GJ, Slaaf DW, Reneman RS: Skeletal muscle microcirculation and changes in transmural and perfusion pressure; in Messmer K, Hammersen F (eds): Skeletal Muscle Microcirculation. Prog Appl Microcirc. Basel, Karger, 1984, vol 5, pp 93–108.

17 Oude Vrielink HHE, Slaaf DW, Tangelder GJ, Reneman RS: Arteriolar and capillay perfusion in rabbit skeletal muscle at rest and during vasodilation. Int J Microcirc Clin Exp 1987;6: 321–332.

18 Sullivan SM, Johnson PC: Effect of oxygen on blood flow autoregulation in cat sartorius muscle. Am J Physiol 1981;241:H807–H815.

Author Index

Subject Index